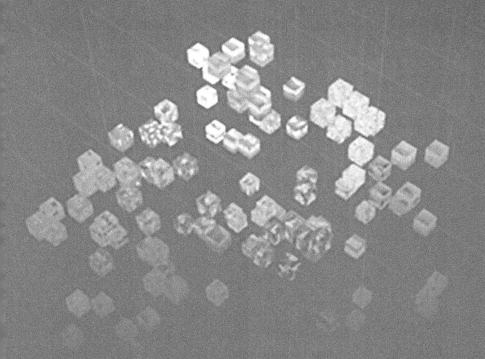

Biomimetics

Biomimetics
Connecting Ecology and Engineering by Informatics

edited by
Akihiro Miyauchi
Masatsugu Shimomura

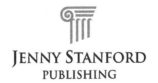

Jenny Stanford
Publishing

Published by

Jenny Stanford Publishing Pte. Ltd.
101 Thomson Road
#06-01, United Square
Singapore 307591

Email: editorial@jennystanford.com
Web: www.jennystanford.com

British Library Cataloguing-in-Publication Data
A catalogue record for this book is available from the British Library.

Biomimetics: Connecting Ecology and Engineering by Informatics
Copyright © 2023 Jenny Stanford Publishing Pte. Ltd.

All rights reserved. This book, or parts thereof, may not be reproduced in any form or by any means, electronic or mechanical, including photocopying, recording or any information storage and retrieval system now known or to be invented, without written permission from the publisher.

ISBN 978-981-4968-10-2 (Hardcover)
ISBN 978-1-003-27717-0 (eBook)

Contents

Preface xv

1. Application of Biomimetics and Public and Industrial Perceptions 1

Yuta Uchiyama, Chika Takatori, and Ryo Kohsaka

1.1	Introduction	2
1.2	Methodology	4
1.3	Museum Visitors Perception 1	6
1.4	Museum Visitors Perception 2	18
1.5	Perception of Industrial Sectors	20
1.6	Comparative Analysis	23

2. Ontology-Enhanced Thesaurus for Promoting Biomimetics Research 25

Riichiro Mizoguchi and Kouji Kozaki

2.1	Introduction		26
2.2	Role of the Knowledge Infrastructure for Biomimetics		28
	2.2.1	Related Work in the Framework of the Design Processes of Biology-Inspired Design	29
	2.2.2	Positioning of OET in the Context of the Whole Design Process	32
	2.2.3	An Envisioned Application	32
		2.2.3.1 How Keyword Explorer works	32
		2.2.3.2 A Motivating Example	34
2.3	Ontology-Enhanced Thesaurus		36
	2.3.1	Characteristics of Biomimetics DBs	36

		2.3.2	Basic Design of a Biomimetics Database Retrieval Scheme	37
		2.3.3	Keyword Exploration as an Independent Task before Issuing Queries to DBs	39
			2.3.3.1 Keyword exploration and missing links	39
			2.3.3.2 Keyword exploration reasoning	40
			2.3.3.3 Two-step help	41
	2.4	Ontologies in OET		42
		2.4.1	Basic Design of Ontologies in OET	42
		2.4.2	Ontology of Function	42
		2.4.3	Concepts other than Function	42
			2.4.3.1 Taxonomy of creatures	43
			2.4.3.2 Properties	44
			2.4.3.3 Living environments	44
			2.4.3.4 The quality of ontologies in OET	45
	2.5	Implementation and Evaluation of a Prototype of Keyword Explorer		45
		2.5.1	Implementation of Keyword Explorer	45
			2.5.1.1 The demo version	46
			2.5.1.2 The prototype version	46
		2.5.2	Preliminary Evaluation Experiment	47
	2.6	Concluding Remarks		48

3. Biomimetics Image Retrieval Platform for Bridging Different Study Fields   **53**

Miki Haseyama and Takahiro Ogawa

3.1	Introduction		54
3.2	Background for New Image Retrieval Platform		56
	3.2.1	Need for an Image Retrieval Scheme in Biomimetics Studies	56
	3.2.2	Image Retrieval Based on a Visualization Technique	56
3.3	Biomimetics Image Retrieval Platform		59

	3.3.1	Algorithm in Our Retrieval Platform	59
	3.3.2	Functions Equipped in the Biomimetics Image Retrieval Platform	60
	3.3.3	Inter-field Similarities Discovered by Our Platform	65
3.4	Conclusions		66

4. Theory of Inventive Problem-Solving Method Applying Biomimetics   **69**

Takeshi Yamauchi, Hidetoshi Kobayashi, and Toru Kobayashi

4.1	Introduction		69
4.2	Current Conditions Regarding Patents for Biomimetics		71
4.3	Engineering Problem Solving Method Applying Biomimetics		72
	4.3.1	TRIZ Method	72
	4.3.2	Bio-TRIZ Method	75
	4.3.3	Examples of Solutions to Technological Contradictions	76
4.4	Database of Inventive Problem-Solving Method Applying Biomimetics		79
	4.4.1	Problem-Oriented Approach-Search from Technical Contradiction Matrix	79
	4.4.2	Function-Oriented Approach-Search from Function	83
	4.4.3	Inventory of Biomimetic Products	84
4.5	A Motivating Example of Database		85
	4.5.1	Problem-Oriented Approach for Windmills	85
	4.5.2	Function-Oriented Approach for Windmills	86
	4.5.3	Inventory of Biomimetic Products for Windmills	87
4.6	Conclusion		88

viii | Contents

5. Urban Planning by Learning from Living Creatures   **91**

Mamoru Taniguchi

5.1	Introduction	91
5.2	Urban Growth and Analogy to Living Creatures	92
5.3	Cities Affected by Lifestyle-Related Diseases	92
	5.3.1 Metabolic Syndrome	92
	5.3.2 Hypertension	94
	5.3.3 Osteoporosis	95
	5.3.4 Cancer	95
5.4	Using Apoptosis in Urban Planning	98
	5.4.1 Two Patterns of Cell Death	98
	5.4.2 Compact Town Development Learned from Apoptosis	98
	5.4.3 Necessity of Reduced Diet	99
	5.4.4 Necessity of District Karte	101
5.5	Concluding Remarks: Thinking about an Evolutionarily Stable Region	102

6. Functional Elucidation of Biological Interactions in Agricultural Ecosystems and the Application of Biomimetics to Plant Protection   **105**

Naoki Mori, Takuma Takanashi, and Hidefumi Mitsuno

6.1	Vibrational Interactions in Beetles and Bugs and Applications in Plant Protection	106
	6.1.1 Background	106
	6.1.2 Vibrational Interactions in Beetles and Bugs	106
	6.1.3 Vibrational Senses	108
	6.1.4 Application of Vibrations in Plant Protection	109
6.2	Contribution of Soybean Leaf Trichomes to the Resistance of *Spodoptera Litura*	112
	6.2.1 Background	112
	6.2.2 Preference Change with and without Soybean Leaf Trichomes	112

6.2.3	Chemical Analysis of Trichome Components	114
6.2.4	Observation and Measurement of Trichome Physical Parameters	115
6.2.5	Discussion	116

6.3	Insect Pheromone Communication	118
6.3.1	Background	118
6.3.2	Reception of Pheromones	119

7. Anti-Biofouling Effects against Sessile Organisms of Soft Materials 129

Takayuki Murosaki

7.1	Introduction	129
7.2	Barnacles	130
7.3	Anti-Biofouling Effects of Soft Materials	132
7.4	Anti-Biofouling Effects of Hydrogels inthe Ocean	136
7.5	Barnacle Growth Inhibition Effects of Soft Materials	138
7.6	Anti-Barnacle Settlement Activity of Microstructured Silicone Elastomers	140
7.7	Conclusion	143

8. Biomimetic Devices by Nano/Micro Processing 149

Seiji Aoyagi, Masato Suzuki, Tomokazu Takahashi, and Takeshi Ito

8.1	Introduction	149
8.2	Fusion of MEMS with Ultra-High-Precision Three-Dimensional Processing	150
8.3	Microneedles for Drawing Blood by Mimicking Mosquitoes	154
8.3.1	Introduction	154
8.3.2	Structure of the Mosquito Needle and the Stinging Motion	155
8.3.3	Manufacture of a Microneedle by Ultra-High-Precision Three-Dimensional Laser Lithography	156

x | Contents

8.3.3.1 Manufacture of a set of three needles to mimic the labrum and two maxillae of a mosquito 157

8.3.3.2 Proposal for needles in which two split-in-half needles are combined 158

8.3.3.3 Manufacture of split-in-half microneedles and evaluation of the piercing and blood-drawing functions 159

8.3.4 Manufacture of a Microneedle Using a Femtosecond Laser 161

8.3.4.1 Hollow needle mimicking the labrum 162

8.3.4.2 Plate-shaped needle having a protrusion with a jagged edge 162

8.3.4.3 Comparison with the proboscis of a mosquito 162

8.3.4.4 Performance evaluation 162

8.4 Vacuum Suction Gripper That Mimics the Octopus Acetabulum 163

8.4.1 Introduction 163

8.4.2 Principle and Structure 164

8.4.3 Gripper Manufacture and Gripping Experiment 165

8.4.3.1 Semispherical gripper with multiple acetabula 166

8.4.3.2 One-acetabulum gripper with a bellows structure 168

8.5 An Antibacterial Nanosurface Mimicking Cicada's Wing Using Biomimetics 170

8.5.1 Introduction 170

8.5.2 Observational Results of Cicada Wings and Manufacturing of a Sample 171

8.5.3 Evaluation of Antibacterial Characteristics 172

| | 8.5.4 | Results | 173 |

8.5.4 Results   173

8.6 Fine Protrusions that Mimic the Footpads of Gecko   174

    8.6.1 Introduction   174

    8.6.2 Measuring the Adhesive Area of the Footpad of Gecko   174

    8.6.3 Adsorption Strength Measurement Experiment   175

    8.6.4 Manufacture of an Adsorption Device Using a Three-Dimensional Laser Lithography and Transfer by UV Nano-Imprinting   177

8.7 A Robot Hand That Mimics the Fingers of a Tree Frog   177

    8.7.1 Introduction   177

    8.7.2 Gripping Strategy   178

    8.7.3 Hand Configuration   179

8.8 Conclusion   182

9. Structural Color in Biomimetics   187

Akira Saito

9.1 Introduction   187

9.2 Optical Principles   188

    9.2.1 Principles for Structural Color   188

    9.2.2 Types of Structural Color   191

9.3 Applications of Structural Color   192

    9.3.1 Advantages of Structural Color   192

    9.3.2 Various Artificial Approaches   193

9.4 "Single Colored" Structural Color: *Morpho* Butterfly   196

    9.4.1 Principles of the Morpho-color   196

    9.4.2 How to Reproduce the Morpho-color?   198

    9.4.3 Another Approach to the *Morpho*-color   200

9.5 New Applications of *Morpho*-Color   201

9.6 Summary   203

10. Wetting Phenomena on Structured Surfaces: Contact Angle, Pinning, Rolling and Bouncing

Hiroyuki Mayama

10.1	Introduction	207
10.2	Equilibrium Contact Angle, Wenzel State and Cassie-Baxter State	208
10.3	Contact Angle: Thermodynamics of Static Wetting Phenomena	210
10.4	Pinning Effect	213
10.5	Lotus Effect	215
10.6	Bouncing Raindrops on Lotus Leaf: Laplace Pressure and Bouncing Phenomena in Dynamic Wetting of Macroscopic Droplets	220
	10.6.1 Laplace Pressure Generated by Surface Structures	222
	10.6.2 Dynamic Pressure	225
	10.6.3 Bouncing Conditions of Macroscopic Droplets and Importance of Standing Angle and Length of Actual Surface Structures	225
	10.6.4 Summary for Bouncing Behaviors of Macroscopic Droplets on Structured Surfaces	229
10.7	Bouncing Phenomena of Smaller Droplets on Structured Surface: Restitution Coefficient	230
10.8	Conclusion	238

11. Powdered Pressure-Sensitive Adhesives Developed Based on Biomimetics

Syuji Fujii and Shin-ichi Akimoto

11.1	Introduction	243
11.2	What are Liquid Marbles?	244
11.3	Liquid Marbles Fabricated by Aphids	245
11.4	Development of PowderedPressure-Sensitive Adhesives	250
11.5	Conclusions	254

Contents | **xiii**

12. Fabrication of Artificial Melanin-Based Structural Color Materials through Biomimetic Design **261**

Michinari Kohri

12.1 Introduction 261

12.2 Structural Colors Found in Nature 262

12.2.1 Role of Melanin in Structural Coloration 262

12.2.2 Melanin and Polydopamine 263

12.3 Structural Coloration by Assembly of Colloidal Particles 264

12.4 Structural Color Materials from Artificial Melanin Particles 265

12.4.1 Structural Coloration from Polydopamine Particles 265

12.4.2 Structural Coloration by Core–Shell Particles with Polydopamine as the Shell Layer 266

12.4.2.1 Particle design 266

12.4.2.2 High-visibility structural coloration 267

12.4.2.3 Effect of assembled structures on coloration 269

12.4.2.4 Effect of compositions on coloration 270

12.4.2.5 Effect of particle shapes on coloration 271

12.4.2.6 Application as coloring materials 272

12.5 Structural Coloration by Black Additives 274

12.6 Perspectives 274

13. Study of Bile Duct Stent Having Antifouling Properties Using Biomimetics Technique **279**

Atsushi Sekiguchi

13.1 Introduction 280

13.2 Biomimetics Technologies 282

13.3 Biliary Stents with Antifouling Properties 284

13.4	Production of Mold with Nanohole Structures Based on Snail Shell Surface Structures	286
13.5	Producing Antifouling Sheets for Stents	286
13.6	Fabrication of Biliary Stent and Liquid Passage Test	288
13.7	In vivo Study	291
	13.7.1 Overview of in vivo Study	291
	13.7.2 In vivo Study Procedure	291
	13.7.3 Results of Animal Testing	292
13.8	Summary	294

14. Biomimetic Designed Surfaces for Growth Suppression of Biofilm-Inspired Sharkskin Denticles — **297**

Mariko Miyazaki and Akihiro Miyauchi

14.1	Introduction	297
14.2	Concept of Biofilm Growth Suppression	301
14.3	Preparation for the Culture Test of Bacteria	303
	14.3.1 Fabrication of Test Sample	303
	14.3.2 Method of Bacterial Culture	305
	14.3.3 Bacterial Culture Conditions	308
	14.3.4 Method of Coverage of Bacteria Quantification	309
14.4	Evaluation of Antibacterial Effect by Biomimetics	310
14.5	Summary	312

Index — 317

Preface

Advances in rapid information technology make it possible to find scientific truths inductively in cyber-space, and this kind of research method is spreading worldwide as a fourth science. On the other hand, living things have undergone numerous trials and errors in the process of evolution, and species acquired the optimum mechanism matching to the global environment. Therefore, the functions of living matters are thought of as obtained by data-driven induction method, and biomimetics is a nature-inspired inductive method.

This book presents contributions from cutting-edge researchers on informatics, ecosystem, and materials. Among the topics covered in this book, a broad range of readers will find the content related to the areas of their interests. The chapters have been organized as follows. Chapters 1 to 4 cover informatics, Chapters 5 to 7 cover ecosystem, and Chapters 8 to 14 cover materials and devices. We hope this book will provide an opportunity to expand readers' ideas for sustainable society.

We thank the chapter contributors, who are lecturers at NBCI (Nanotechnology Business Creation Initiative) seminars, and especially thank Mrs. Masaki Aoki and Masahiro Imaizumi for arranging these seminars.

Akihiro Miyauchi and Masatsugu Shimomura
2022

Chapter 1

Application of Biomimetics and Public and Industrial Perceptions

Yuta Uchiyama,[a] Chika Takatori,[b] and Ryo Kohsaka[c]

[a]*Graduate School of Human Development and Environment, Kobe University, Kobe City, Hyogo 657-8501, Japan*
[b]*Graduate School of Design, Kyushu University, Fukuoka City, Fukuoka 815-8540, Japan*
[c]*Graduate School of Environmental Studies, Nagoya University, Nagoya City, Aichi 464-8601, Japan*

kohsaka@hotmail.com

This chapter introduces the results of a questionnaire survey on the awareness of biomimetic technology to provide implications for social implementation of biomimetics. There is a common trend among survey results, which is that medical industry is expected as promising application industry of biomimetics. The results show that biomimetic technology application is in the process of shifting to the sub-cellular size and to the larger-scale application. The information sharing, such as exhibition of biomimetics, can influence the respondents' perceptions, and there is a room for further research on communication methods among stakeholders in the process of social implementation of biomimetics.

Biomimetics: Connecting Ecology and Engineering by Informatics
Edited by Akihiro Miyauchi and Masatsugu Shimomura
Copyright © 2023 Jenny Stanford Publishing Pte. Ltd.
ISBN 978-981-4968-10-2 (Hardcover), 978-1-003-27717-0 (eBook)
www.jennystanford.com

1.1 Introduction

Intergovernmental science-policy Platform on Biodiversity and Ecosystem Services (IPBES) plans to conduct an assessment on "business and biodiversity" and scoping process is likely to be initiated in near future (Fig. 1.1). The assessments are likely to include the linkages of operational business impacts in a negative manner to biodiversity and ecosystems. Simultaneously, there are potentials that the positive impacts may also be highlighted from biodiversity and ecosystems (or Natures Contribution to People [NCPs]) to Research and Development (R&D).

Biomimetics is one of the leading areas where such positive impacts are observed and appreciated in a concrete manner as a benefit to the society and human well-being, particularly for the field of R&D in manufacturing sectors (possible comparable to pollutions for agricultural productions). Conservation efforts to biodiversity is frequently met with questions of significance and relevance of biodiversity to human well-being and impacts to society. Understanding perceptions and expectations of biomimetics are, thus, one of the most crucial, if the most crucial question for the biodiversity conservation and sustainable use efforts.

There are a number of recent developments related to biomimetics and business. With the proposal and initiative of French organization, expert committees are established for biodiversity under the International Organization for Standardization (ISO) framework. In June 2020, member body voted in favor to approve the creation of a new Technical Committee on Biodiversity, and Allocates the secretariat to AFNOR (ISO TECHNICAL MANAGEMENT BOARD RESOLUTION 47/2020).

Both moves in IPBES and ISO are ongoing and it is not easily foreseen what will happen there. Yet, there are some past lessons and experiences accumulated in the field of biomimetics. One of the authors (Kohsaka) in this chapter has been active in TC 266/WG4 as convener together with other experts (Prof. Shimomura, Dr. Hirasaka, Dr. Kobayashi, Dr. Yamauchi) in this volume.

As such, there are needs to understand the trends and status of perceptions for both in industries and the public.

Reflecting such emerging changes in the field, we aim to highlight the perceptions, expectations and gaps or potential rooms for improvements for biomimetics for lay people, business sectors and scientists alike.

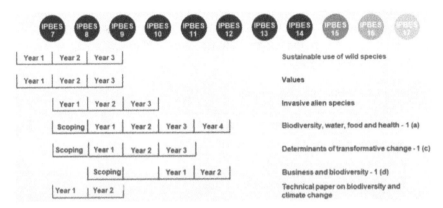

Figure 1.1 Plan of IPBES assessments (*Source*: IPBES).

To facilitate the social implementation of biomimetics, an understanding of public and industrial perceptions of biomimetics is needed. Existing studies indicate that social values of the ecosystem in environmental management reflect public perceptions [1]. Regarding the social implementation of biotechnology, negative public perceptions may be hindrances of the growth of the related market [2]. Still, if the relevant information is provided to stakeholders, their perceptions can be changed [3]. The development of technologies is dynamically changing. Given the dynamic characteristics of the technology development and public perceptions, the latest perceptions need to be detected to facilitate the social implementation of technologies.

Participation of various stakeholders is required in the process of social implementation [4]. Identifying the perceptions of various stakeholders on biomimetics can contribute to its social implementation.

In the following sections, methodology of survey and survey results of museum visitors and private company staff members are provided.

1.2 Methodology

We conducted questionnaire survey to museum visitors and private company staff members in Japan. In the questionnaire survey, respondents were asked to choose the three most promising technologies from 20 practical technologies based on biomimetics (Table 1.1). The identical classification items "field of application" (technical field to which biomimetics is applied), which is used in the Japan Patent Office (JPO) study [5], were used in the surveys.

Table 1.1 Promising technologies

Hydrophilic & hydrophobic material (Material)
Structural coloring material (Material)
Adhesive material (Material)
Medical & biocompatible material (Material)
Optical material (Material)
Battery & semiconductor material (Material)
High strength & toughness material (Material)
Self-repairing material (Material)
Low resistance & friction material (Material)
Antifouling material (Material)
Others (Material)
Lightweight (Structure)
Low resistance & friction (Structure)
Others (Structure)
Robot (Machine)
Sensor (Machine)
Control (Machine)
Actuator (Machine)
Product process (Machine)

In Table 1.1, "Material" refers to various functional materials such as hydrophilic and hydrophobic materials, structural coloring materials, adhesive materials, and molecules such as artificial enzymes. "Structure" is a macro structure including a car imitating a boxfish. "Machine" is robotics technologies for biomimetics. "Process" refers to a manufacturing process applying biomineralization and a biotemplate. "Production Process", which is the process of material production or structure formation of an organism, is included in the items JPO [5].

Table 1.2 shows applied promising industries that are commonly used for this study and past studies of the JPO. We asked respondents to choose the three most promising application industries from 31 practical industry fields for biomimetics.

Table 1.2 Promising industries

Artificial organ (Medical)
Cell culture material (Medical)
DDS (Medical)
Surgical glue (Medical)
Medical apparatus (Medical)
Others (Medical)
Power generation apparatus (Environment & energy)
Artificial photosynthesis (Environment & energy)
Water treatment (Environment & energy)
Others (Environment & energy)
Optical communication (Communication)
Others (Communication)
Disaster rescue robot (Safe & secure)
Detection system (Safe & secure)
Others (Safe & secure)
Culture implement (Agriculture, forestry & fisheries)
Insect pest control (Agriculture, forestry & fisheries)
Others (Agriculture, forestry & fisheries)
Transportation equipment material (Transportation)
Transportation equipment parts (Transportation)
Traffic control (Transportation)

(Continued)

Table 1.2 (*Continued*)

Others (Transportation)
Electrical appliance & optics parts (Consumer products)
Fiber material (Consumer products)
Cosmetics (Consumer products)
Daily necessities (Consumer products)
Others (Consumer products)
Construction material (Construction)
Others (Construction)
Others

1.3   Museum Visitors Perception 1

In "Insect Exhibition" (period: July 13th to 8th October 2018) by the National Museum of Nature and Science, we conducted surveys in two days (dates: 10th and 20th August). We obtained answers from the visitors to the exhibitions as respondents (n = 310). The percentage of gender is roughly balance with 45% female and 54% male. The age group was 27% for children under 10 years old, 25% for teens, 12% for 30s, and 40s were 21%. 35% were with children, 41% were adults, and 14% were with their friends (Fig. 1.2). There were larger portion of family visitors given the characteristics of the exhibitions. Looking at the percentage by occupations, students and office workers accounted for 57%. As for the profile for the place residence, 50% of the houses were in urban areas, 43% were in new residential areas, and 8% were in rural areas, mainly from urban areas and new residential areas. As for the frequency of visits, the numbers were generally low, such as "1 to 5 times a year", "once every few years", or "almost never", accounting for 91% of the total. This implies that the exhibition was potentially effective in attracting layers of visitors who would not visit the exhibitions in ordinary circumstances.

We asked whether the visitors knew "biomimetic technology" and to what extent. The majority responded negatively that they were not aware of the technology and answers of "do not know" was 211 (69%). Alternatively, the awareness was rather limited to 25 (8%) who responded "I know, I also know specific products and technologies." Less than quarter, or 71 (23%), responded that "I have heard the name" (Fig. 1.3). It was identified that the general recognition was not high even those who are motivated to visit the exhibitions and potentially interested in the insects than general public.

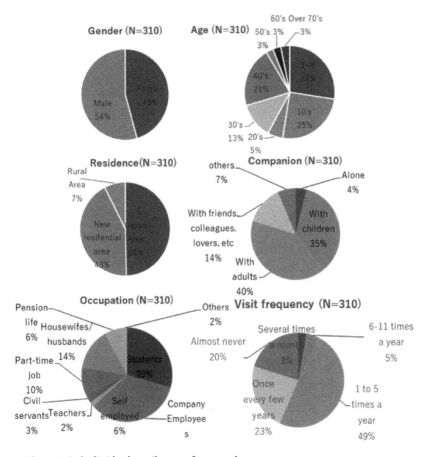

Figure 1.2 Individual attributes of respondents.

Next, regarding the promising applied technologies and applied industries in biomimetic technology, the most promising ones and the top three respectively were asked to the respondents.

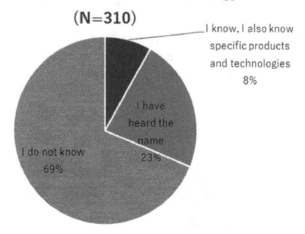

Figure 1.3 The answers on whether they know "biomimetic technology".

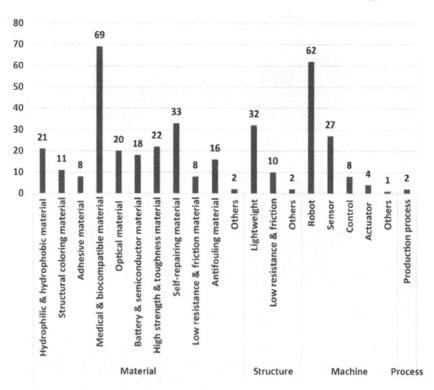

Figure 1.4 Expected application technology.

As a result of applied technology, 69 people (22%) thought that "Medical bio compatible material (Material)" was promising and 62 people (20%) thought "Robot (Machine)"was promising. It became clear that they were the largest values. "Self-repairing material (Material)" was 33 (11%), "Lightweight (Structure)" was 32 (10%), and "Sensor (Machine)" was 27 (9%) (Fig. 1.4).

For the applied technology, we analyzed the trends and percentages of promising technologies based on gender, age, residence, and household status. As for gender, female interviewees tended to choose following items as promising technology than male; "Medical and biocompatible material (Material)", "Robot (Machine)", and "Lightweight (Structure)". Alternatively, male respondents tended to opt for "High-strength and toughness material (Material)", "Battery and semiconductor material (Material), "Self-repairing material (Material)", and "Sensor (Process)" (Fig. 1.5).

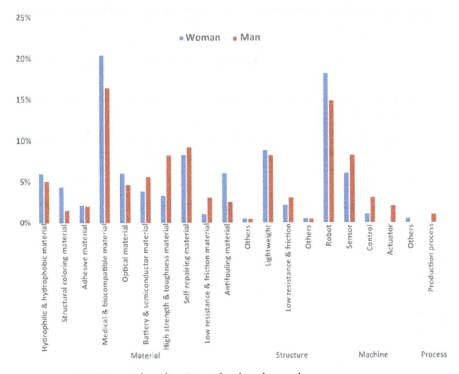

Figure 1.5 Expected application technology by gender.

In a similar vein, we analyzed the trends by individual age groups (Fig. 1.6). As general trends, it turned out that the age groups with high hopes and interests were different for each application.

For the group children under 10 years of age thought that "Medical and biocompatible material (Material)" and "Robot (Machine)" were the most promising applied technologies. Uniquely for this age group, "Structure" group was promising was low at 0%, indicating that the fields that seemed promising for them were biased within the scope of their interests. These may have certain implications for future exhibitions and rooms to evoking interests in environmental educations for such fields. As for the teens, wider variety of fields seemed promising, implying expansions of their areas of interests. For those in their 20s, "Hydrophilic and hydrophobic material (Material)" and "Self-repairing material (Material)" were more likely to be promising. "Antifouling material (Material)" was most frequently chosen by the respondents in their 30s. It was "Self-repairing material (Material)" for the elderly in their 70s, "Lightweight (Structure)" for those in the 60s. It could be said that there are different trends for children under 10 but the "Medical and biocompatible material (Material)", "Robot (Machine)" and "Self-repairing material" are generally the technologies that are chosen as promising technologies for wide range of age groups.

We analyzed the tendency by residence areas (Fig. 1.7). For those living in rural areas, "Medical and biocompatible material (Material)" had a high percentage. Alternatively, "Robot (Machine)" had a higher value for those living in urban areas. In rural areas, a high percentage of people thought that "Self-repairing material (Material)" and "Lightweight (Structure)" were promising. This is mainly due to the overlap with the age group that those living in rural areas are composed of elderly people in their 60s and 70s. In contrast, the percentage of people in new residential areas tended to opt for "Hydrophilic and hydrophobic material (Material)", "Antifouling material (Material)", and "High-strength and toughness material (Material)" than other groups. This is, again, due to age factor that the new residential areas are composed of young people (20's or 30's).

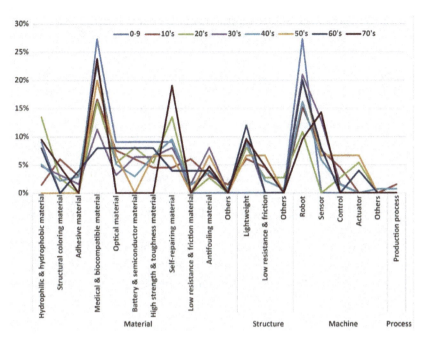

Figure 1.6 Expected application technology by age.

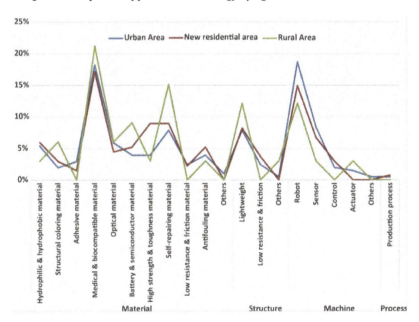

Figure 1.7 Expected application technology by residence.

We further analyzed the trends by companion status (Fig. 1.8). Those respondents who came "with adults" tended to opt for "Medical and biocompatible material (Material)" and "Robot (Machine)" as promising technology. This was a similar tendency according to age, which showed the results from the young people under 10. Furthermore, the respondents who were accompanied "with children" tended to choose "Self-repairing material (Material)" and "Lightweight (Structure)" in addition to the "Medical and biocompatible material (Material)" and "Robot (Machine)". From the results, a typical portfolio would be elderly who came from rural areas with their grandchildren and parents in their twenties and thirties in the new urban area answered in the manner.

On the other hand, it was found that those who came "alone" thought that "High-strength and toughness material (Material)" was the most promising, which tended to be different from other respondents.

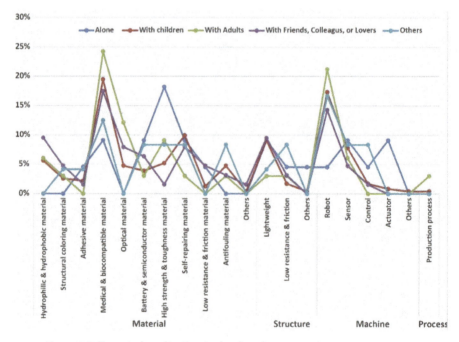

Figure 1.8 Expected application technology by companion.

In the following section, we provide the results of promising fields or "application industries with high expectations". We first simply show the tabulation of applied industries with high expectations before considering other factors. From the results, "Medical" field was chosen as most frequently followed by "Artificial organ (Medical)" with 55 people (18%), "Cell culture material (Medical)" with 48 people (15%), "Medical apparatus" (Medical) with 36 people (12%) (Fig. 1.9).

The following field was "Insect pest control (Agriculture, forestry and fisheries)" by 32 people (10%) and "Disaster rescue robot (Safe and secure)" by 30 people (10%). Those who thought that "Medical and biocompatible material (Material)" and "Robot (Machine)" were promising in applied technology were also interested the related fields in applied industries which is an understandable trend.

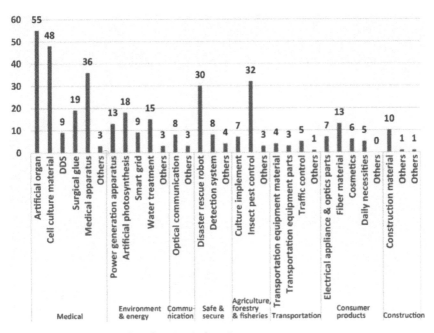

Figure 1.9 Expected application industries.

We summarize the relation between the chosen applied industries and the promising attributes of the respondents (gender, age, residence, occupation, accompanying persons).

Leading portion (roughly 15%) of both of male and female chose "Artificial organ (Medical)" as promising field. There were certain differences in gender and females tend to prefer with higher frequency the "Cell culture material (Medical)" and "Insect pest control (Agriculture, forestry and fisheries)", "Disaster rescue robot (Safe and secure)", "Artificial photosynthesis (Environment and energy)" as promising fields. For male respondents, it was "Medical Apparatus (Medical)", "Water treatment (Environment and energy)", and "Fiber material (Consumer products)" (Fig. 1.10).

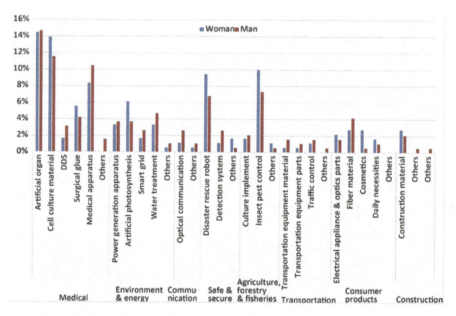

Figure 1.10 Application industries by gender.

There were trends by age groups; respondents under the age of 10 had the tendency to choose fields of "Artificial organ (Medical)", "Cell culture material (Medical)" and "DDS (Medical)" as promising fields, all above 25%. Similar to applied technology, the range of answers was widespread in the teens and above. For those in their 20s, "Medical apparatus (Medical)" and "Insect pest control (Agriculture, forestry and fisheries)" were 15% and 13%, respectively, showing high rates of preferences. For those in their 30s, "Disaster rescue robot (Safe and Secure)" showed a particularly high interest of 10% or more. For those in the

50s, "Water treatment (Environment and energy)" was high at 10% or more, while those in their 70s, "Water treatment (Environment and energy)" and "Detection system (Safe and secure)" were both 10%. This is due to increasing interest in environmental/energy issues and safety/security issues as the age rises. As seen above, certain trends were identified the applied industry according to the age groups (Fig. 1.11).

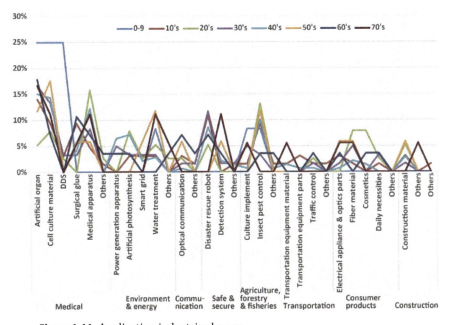

Figure 1.11 Application industries by age.

We provide the trends based on the types of residences (urban and rural). The ration of "Artificial organ (Medical)" and "Disaster rescue robot (Safe and secure)" were significantly higher for those from urban areas and new residential areas compared to rural areas (Fig. 1.12).

It is partially due to the growing interest in countermeasures against the increasing natural disasters in urban areas in recent years at the time such as typhoons and other disasters. For those from rural areas, such as "Cell culture material (Medical)" and "Medical apparatus (Medical)" in the medical field were more frequently chosen as expected application fields. For the field of

16 | *Application of Biomimetics and Public and Industrial Perceptions*

"Insect pest control (Agriculture, forestry and fisheries)" had a high proportion of respondents across the residential areas, both in rural, urban areas and also emerging urban areas, indicating widespread expectations across generations.

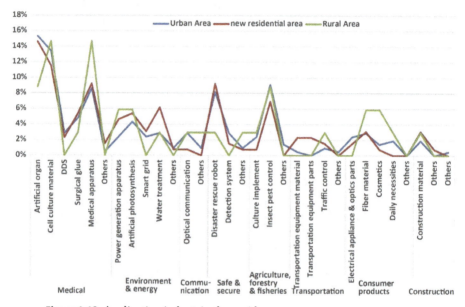

Figure 1.12 Application industries by residence.

We also analyzed the trends by companions of respondents of "expected application industries" (Fig. 1.13). Children accompanied by "adults" had high interests in "Artificial organ (Medical)" which was 20% or more. The option "Insect pest control (Agriculture, forestry and fisheries)" followed with 13%, which were second-highest percentage in all other items. The results were similar with the trends in the age groups of children under 10 to those in their teens. In contrast, for parents and grandparents whose companions were "children" and those whose companions were "friends, colleagues, lovers, etc.", it could be seen that the expectations were diverse and showed no clear trends. Furthermore, respondents who came "alone" thought that "Medical apparatus (Medical)", "Detection system (Safe and secure)", "Traffic control (Transportation)", "Artificial photosynthesis (Environment and energy)", "Fiber material (Consumer products)" were with high expectations, and the group indicated unique tendency from those who visited in a group.

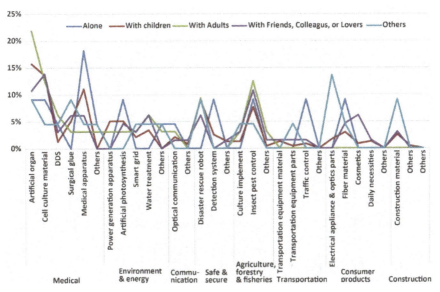

Figure 1.13 Application industries by companion.

Finally, we analyzed the relationship between knowledge of biomimetic technology and applied industries with high prospects and expectations (Fig. 1.14). For those who "know well" about biomimetic technology, the group tended to choose "Medical apparatus (Medical)", "Disaster rescue robot (Robot)", "Smart grid (Environment and energy)" and "Fiber material". High percentage of the people that knew the technology answered that "Consumer products" and "Construction material (Construction)" were fields with high expectations. They may have seen or heard the above knowledge of applied industries before.

In contrast, those who answered "I have heard their name" or "I do not know" thought that "Artificial organ (Medical)" and "Insect pest control (Agriculture, forestry and fisheries)" were particularly chosen as fields with high expectation. It was also found that "Medical apparatus (Medical)" and "Disaster rescue robot (Robot)" had a high proportion in the group.

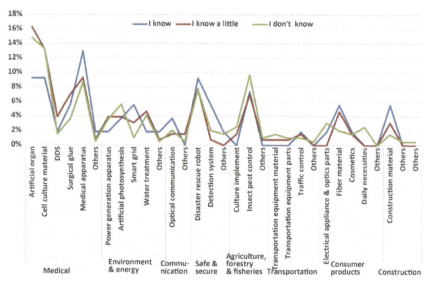

Figure 1.14 Application industries by knowledge of biomimetic technology.

1.4 Museum Visitors Perception 2

We conducted another survey at an exhibition held at the National Museum of Nature and Science, Tokyo in 2016 [6]. Data were collected across holidays and work days; April 29 and May 3 were holidays, and May 2 and June 6 were average workdays. The exhibition was held in collaboration with the research project "Innovative Materials Engineering Based on Biological Diversity" (2012–2016). A growing interest in biomimetics fields has been observed, and exhibiting and sharing the latest biomimetics for visitors at the National Museum of Nature and Science in Tokyo are needed. The results of the project were disseminated to the public in the exhibition.

Responses from 216 museum visitors were collected. The respondents were randomly sampled during the set dates. A relatively large number of responses were collected from those in their teens and 20s. The relatively younger generation respondents are composed of the high school students visiting the museum on school trips or group visits of university students.

We collected 88 responses at the gate of exhibition room from respondents whose ages are between 30 and 50. They tended to visit the museum with their families.

Figure 1.15 shows the respondents' perceptions of practical technology. It reveals that the most promising technologies were in the fields of molecules and materials. The highest percentage of respondents indicated biocompatible medical materials (39%) as a promising technology, followed by self-repair materials, and hydrophobic and hydrophilic materials. The percentages of robots (23%) and sensor technology (21%) were highest in the mechanical engineering field. In the structural field, weight reduction technology (18%) was the most expected technology.

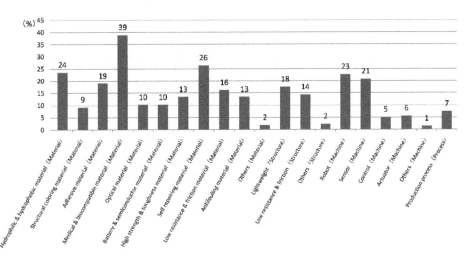

Figure 1.15 Promising technologies.

Figure 1.16 provides the results of respondents' perceptions on the promising industry for application of biomimetics. The most popular industry was the medical field, followed by industries related to the environment or energy. As for individual industries, the most selected application industry was artificial organs in medical fields, followed by medical apparatus and cell culture materials. For the environment and energy fields, power facilities were expected with a ratio of more than 15%.

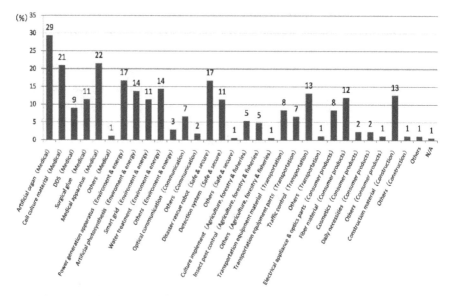

Figure 1.16 Promising industries.

1.5 Perception of Industrial Sectors

We conducted the online survey of employees from private companies in 2016 [7]. The survey period is from 27th to 28th December. The total number of respondents was 276. From each designated industrial sector shown in Table 1.3, 20 people were targeted. The respondents are staff members from companies in the manufacturing and service sectors. The gender ratio of the respondents is not balanced because of the actual composition of the staff working in the field or sector in Japan. The manufacturing sector includes industries directly related to biomimetic technologies. The service sector including the financial services industry was considered as one of the stakeholders of the R&D and social implementation.

As for the applied technologies, Materials were most expected technologies and considered the most promising technologies (Fig. 1.17). Three applied technologies including Medical and biocompatible material (Material), Hydrophilic and hydrophobic material (Material), and Self-repairing material (Material) were tended to be chosen by respondents as promising technologies. These three technologies are considered as conventional biomimetics technologies among the respondents. For instance, hydrophobic material inspired by the lotus-leaf is relatively popular and common, and this fact can be a reason why the percentage for hydrophobic material is high among the listed applied technologies.

Table 1.3 Industrial sectors

Construction
Textiles and Apparels
Chemicals
Pharmaceutical, Cosmetics
Rubber Products
Glass and Ceramics Products
Iron and Steel
Nonferrous Metals
Metal Products
Machinery
Semiconductor, Electrical Equipment
Transportation Equipment
Precision Instruments
Banks (City Bank) (Local Bank)
Securities
Electric Power and Gas, Energy

The sub-cellular scale technologies are expected to be applied technologies of biomimetics. On the other hand, there is little expectation from the Machine field, which has relatively larger-scale technologies. The fact that the trend for biomimetic technology is in the process of shifting to the sub-cellular size seems to be reflected in the result [8]. Considering the result of this survey, implementing the knowledge transfer and experience sharing among stakeholders who focus on biomimetic technology across different spatial scales to facilitate the development and social implementation of biomimetics is needed. The experience in the development of larger-scale biomimetics is relatively limited as compared with those of nanoscale biomimetics, and such experience needs to be shared among stakeholders.

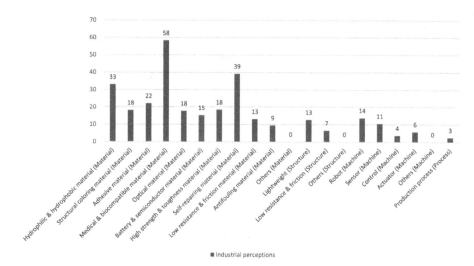

Figure 1.17 Promising technologies.

Regarding the promising industries, the trend that medical fields are expected by the respondents is commonly shown (Fig. 1.18). The trend is relatively obvious compared with other survey results.

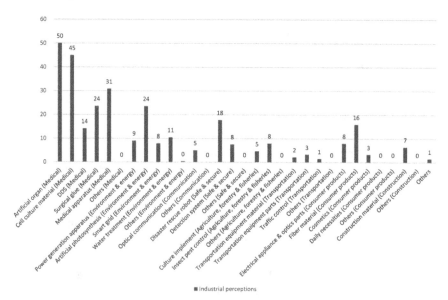

Figure 1.18 Promising industries.

1.6 Comparative Analysis

In this section, public and industrial perceptions are compared using the three survey results. The overall trends are similar in the three survey results (Figures 1.19 and 1.20).

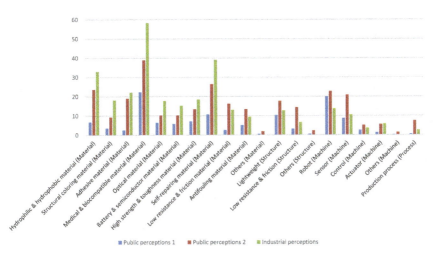

Figure 1.19 Promising technologies.

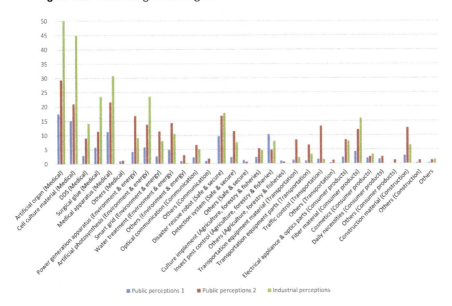

Figure 1.20 Promising industries.

For example, promising applied technologies are the technologies in material fields. Promising industry for which biomimetics can apply is medical industry.

The contents of exhibitions influence public perceptions in certain degree. For example, museum visitors in the insect exhibition tend to choose the insect related technologies and industries. Such patterns of the influence of the information sharing need to be considered in the facilitation of the social implementation of biomimetics. In the future studies, effective and efficient communication methods for stakeholders' participation and collaboration can be analyzed based on the results of this study.

References

1. Ives, C. D., and Kendal, D. (2014). The role of social values in the management of ecological systems. *Journal of Environmental Management*, **144**, 67–72.

2. Brinegar, K., et al. (2017). The commercialization of genome-editing technologies. *Critical Reviews in Biotechnology*, **37**(7), 924-932.

3. Braun, R. (2002). People's concerns about biotechnology: some problems and some solutions. *Journal of Biotechnology*, **98**, 3–8.

4. Tempelman, E., et al. (2015). Biomimicry and cradle to cradle in product design: an analysis of current design practice. *Journal of Design Research*, **13**, 326–344.

5. Japan Patent Office (JPO). (2015). The Reports on Patent Application Trends: Biomimetics.

6. Kohsaka, R. et al. (2017). Public perception and expectations of biomimetics technology: empirical survey of museum visitors in Japan. *Curator: The Museum Journal*, **60**, 427–444.

7. Kohsaka, R., Fujihira, Y., Uchiyama, Y. (2019). Biomimetics for business? Industry perceptions and patent application. *Journal of Science and Technology Policy Management*, **10**, 597–616.

8. Shimomura, M. (2010). The new trends in next generation biomimetics material technology: learning from biodiversity. *Science & Technology Trends Quarterly Review*, **3**, 53–75.

Chapter 2

Ontology-Enhanced Thesaurus for Promoting Biomimetics Research

Riichiro Mizoguchi[a,b] and Kouji Kozaki[c]

[a]*Japan Advanced Institute for Science and Technology,*
1-1 Asahidai, Nomi, Ishikawa 923-1292, Japan
[b]*Laboratory for Applied Ontology,*
ISTC-CNR, Via alla Cascata 56/C, Povo, Trento 38123, Italy
[c]*Faculty of Information and Communication Engineering,*
Osaka Electro-Communication University,
12-16 Hayakocho, Neyagawa-shi, Osaka 572-0837, Japan

mizo@jaist.ac.jp, kozaki@osakac.ac.jp

This chapter discusses Ontology-Enhanced Thesaurus (OET) and Keyword Explorer, which play a role of the knowledge infrastructure for promoting biomimetics research. They support efficient information search by filling the gap between engineering and biology through keyword exploration reasoning based on the biomimetics ontology. The Keyword Explorer provides appropriate keywords with users to help them find information useful for innovative biology-inspired engineering. The prototype of Ontology-Enhanced Thesaurus and Keyword Explorer has been implemented with the prototype ontology and was evaluated through a trial use by 16 companies. The result shows these technologies are promising and expected to promote biomimetics.

Biomimetics: Connecting Ecology and Engineering by Informatics
Edited by Akihiro Miyauchi and Masatsugu Shimomura
Copyright © 2023 Jenny Stanford Publishing Pte. Ltd.
ISBN 978-981-4968-10-2 (Hardcover), 978-1-003-27717-0 (eBook)
www.jennystanford.com

2.1 Introduction

The key to the diffusion of biomimetics is the strongly coordinated efforts among the researchers in biology, and the researchers and engineers in chemistry, physics, and other related disciplines. The most prominent characteristic of biomimetics, when compared with traditional approaches, is the existence of a gap between engineering/technology and biology, which derives the necessity to promote smooth communication between the two parties and to help them find relevant information (see Fig. 2.1). From engineering point of view, we can expect a reasonable contribution to facilitation of developing practical solutions for engineering problems by utilizing the accumulated knowledge in biology. Ontology-Enhanced Thesaurus and Keyword Explorer have been proposed to contribute to filling the gap effectively.

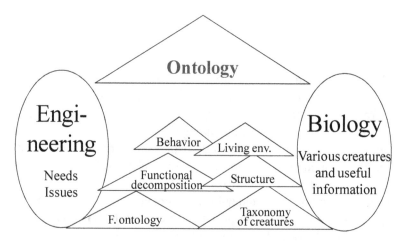

Figure 2.1 Bridging the gap by ontologies.

This chapter describes implemented prototypes of Ontology-Enhanced Thesaurus and Keyword Explorer running on OET. Although we discuss design philosophy of these two, the discussion should be understood as an exposure of the reason why and how they work rather than the guideline for their future mplementation. Ontology is expected to act as a conceptual foundation of the target domain by organizing the related domain knowledge and data for facilitating interoperability among them. This is easily understood when one considers the fact that knowledge and data are equal to what we know about the reality.

Ontology engineering research [19] has been intensively conducted in the last two decades. Several upper ontologies are already available [20–22] and many domain ontologies have been built [33, 34]. Although they work as a kind of knowledge infrastructure, applications developed on top of them have been mainly for metadata of various resources [35] to date. Considering the difficulties for building good ontologies, more appealing applications which deserve the cost of building such ontologies are highly expected.

Although the ontology in OET looks like an ordinary ontology as a kind of ontology mentioned above, it is different from the existing ones in the sense that it is a specialization of such conventional ontologies that are developed for generic purposes or use for metadata. It is built for efficient information search to realize an advanced and a new kind of thesaurus which would facilitate the coordination among the relevant disciplines. In fact, Ontology-Enhanced Thesaurus has been designed for making information search more efficient by filling the gap between engineering and biology (see Fig. 2.1). In order to demonstrate the utility and value of OET, we discuss its example of implementation together with an application program called Keyword Explorer which is an example application running on OET.

We here clarify the relation between the purpose of Working Group (WG)4 of International Standard Organization (ISO)Technical Committees (TC)/266 and OET. WG4 has been established under the name of knowledge infrastructure of biomimetics. OET is an output as the result of our activity under the umbrella of knowledge infrastructure of biomimetics (ISO TC/266). As is discussed in detail in the following sections, OET covers only a portion of it and is roughly composed of an ontology of biomimetics and an application named Keyword Explorer running on it. Readers are recommended to understand Keyword Explorer as a concrete and practical example to exploit the potential utility of the ontology of biomimetics. In spite of our strong belief that the importance of the notion of knowledge infrastructure of biomimetics, we learned it is not well-understood among practitioners. This is partly because why we developed Keyword Explorer for practitioners to convince them of the utility of the ontology of biomimetics.

Let us make another clarification about the relation between OET and a thesaurus. As OET stands for Ontology-Enhanced Thesaurus, readers might be interested in how they collaborate together. The answer to this question is that they work in a loosely coupled manner. That is, OET neither is built in a thesaurus nor is literally built on top of a thesaurus. We could say that these two works almost independently of each other. So, OET can work with any thesaurus in a harmonic manner to effectively enhance its capacity. The details are discussed in Sections 2.2.3.2 and 2.3.3.3.

The structure of this chapter is as follows. In Section 2.2, after a brief overview of the current state of the art of tools and systems in biomimetics, we position OET in the related work, and then we overview OET and Keyword Explorer. In Section 2.3, OET is discussed together with its design rationale. In-depth discussion on the implemented ontology in OET is done in Section 2.4. In order to get feedback from readers about the implemented prototype of Keyword Explorer, how to run and evaluate it are described in Section 2.5 followed by the future direction of OET in Section 2.6 on concluding remarks.

2.2 Role of the Knowledge Infrastructure for Biomimetics

The flow chart of a bionic development process is understood as composed of the following eight phases: Development of ideas, Analysis, Analogy/Abstraction, Project/design of experiments, Experiments and calculations, Prototype construction/ manufacturing, Application tests and Overall evaluation. Among standards established in TC266, ISO18457 and ISO18458 define and exposit the phases from "Analysis" to "Overall evaluation." And ISO18459 covers the phases from "Project/design of experiment" to "Prototype construction/manufacturing." Although the activity of WG4 covers the phases from "Development of ideas" to "Analogy/abstraction", OET described in this chapter covers mainly the first phase of "Development of ideas" and is composed of an ontology and Keyword Explorer. The latter is a tool for helping concept formation running on the former intended to demonstrate its utility.

2.2.1 Related Work in the Framework of the Design Processes of Biology-Inspired Design

There are quite a few systems/tools for supporting innovative design based on biomimetics or Biology-Inspired Design (BID). We classify them according to two dimensions such as the phase of the targeted design process and the degree of automation of the provided support. The design process is here divided into two phases such as concept formation and the analysis & analogy/ abstraction. In the former phase, information retrieval from databases is the key activity, and in the latter, problem solving is the key activity. Researchers have put their effort in making the communication between engineering and biology smoothly in either phase. The other dimension, the degree of intelligence, is about how much the system/tool can help engineers proactively and has two values such as high and low intelligence. According to these four values, existing systems/tools can be classified into four kinds as shown in Table 2.1.

Table 2.1 Classification of existing systems/tools

	High intelligence	Low intelligence
Concept formation (Idea creation) phase	Vincent [44] OET	AskNature [23] Jacobs [31][38], Shu[25] Nagel [37], Cheong [14]
Analysis and Analogy/abstraction phases	Chakrabarti [28] Vattam [30] Goel [13][41] Hollermann [32]	BioTRIZ [24]

Chakrabarti [28] develops a system automated analogical search of relevant ideas based on a generic model for representing causality of natural and artificial systems. It helps to develop novel, analogical ideas for solving design problems using inspiration from both natural and artificial worlds. Vattam [30] analyzes an intricate episode of biologically inspired design in terms of Why, What, How and When questions of analogy. The analysis provides certain patterns of distribution of analogies and a content theory of creative analogies in biologically inspired innovative design.

Goel's system, named DANE (Design Analogy to Nature Engine) [13, 41], is a sophisticated AI system and helps engineers conduct Bio-Inspired Design. The system has four primary components: (1) to facilitate biologically inspired design activity, (2) cognitive research platform, (3) augmented intelligence platform and (4) structured representation development. It seems to have a difficulty in scalability because all the relevant and necessary resources for inspiration from biology have to be prepared in the system in advance.

Hollermann [32] develops a biomimetic methodology and tool for supporting creativity in product innovation based on a general bionic concept including a detailed guideline. It supports the identification of biological models through the iSEE (iterative semantic examination) process.

BioTRIZ [24] is a specialization of TRIZ technology developed for innovative design in engineering [36] to enable BID. It is a long-term project and is intended to help engineers to perform BID by suggesting possible solution candidates which biological organisms have already solved. It is originated from the analysis of successful patents based on scientific and empirically derived methodology. The BioTRIZ consists of a set of tools and supports the users to solve practically any problem using various rules and techniques. It is a truly ambitious project.

Vincent [44] develops an ontology for biomimetics focusing on the trade-off as a central concept to bridge the gap between biology and problem solving in engineering. The concept of the trade-off is defined using the method of the TRIZ Contradiction Matrix. The ontology can identify trade-offs, suggest biological analogues and the principles for BID.

AskNatrue [23] is a comprehensive database of several kinds of useful resources of BID. It consists of four primary types of interconnected information: (1) biological strategies, (2) inspired ideas related to BID, (3) resources for learning/teaching BID, and (4) collections of themed clusters of them, curated by the users. BioM Innovation Database [31, 38] is a database for success stories as case studies of BID with sophisticated statistical analyses so that it supports the users to research and develop detailed case studies. Each case included in the database is linked to information such as patents, descriptions on product and biological model, analysis of biomimetic criteria and classification, relevant sources and so on. Although either one provides useful information, they are essentially databases and for human consumption. More proactive help by the system is found in several papers by Shu's group based on functional basis [25, 42, 43].

The closest research to Keyword Explorer on OET is found in the work Nagel [37] and Cheong [14] conducted by Stone and Shu's groups [25, 42, 43]. Their main purpose is to fill the gap between functional terms used in engineering and biology. They employ the functional basis [1] which is widely accepted as a standardized representation of engineering product functionality in USA. The keywords based on functional basis are expected to work as a thesaurus to help engineers find biological analogies relevant to their design problems. They actually built a thesaurus for translating engineering functional terms to biological functional terms. These functional terms enable engineers to identify biologically meaningful keywords therefore it helps them retrieve and apply relevant analogies. In spite of the similarity of the goal to OET, however, their work is different from OET in two respects. One is that it only deals with functional terms, whereas OET covers organisms, features, living environments, structure in an ontology as well as functions, and the other is that they mainly provide biological functional terms for information retrieval, while the Keyword Explorer directly provides candidates organisms as possible solutions on the basis of association-based inference on OET.

2.2.2 Positioning of OET in the Context of the Whole Design Process

The most important reason why the knowledge infrastructure for biomimetics is necessary is already stated in the Section 3.5 of "The communication process in biomimetics" in the VDI 6220 Biomimetics – Conceptions and strategy differences between bionic and conventional methods/products. As the biomimetics is a cross-disciplinary endeavor, it is crucial for all relevant disciplines to exchange their accumulated knowledge and ideas for biomimetic discoveries and developments. Each discipline has developed its unique set of concepts, words, and their meanings and usages. Without a proper translation mechanism, it is obvious that the communication among the disciplines will be hindered.

While researchers and engineers go through the above phases, they go forward three steps. The first step is to identify the problem to be solved, and find the biological models as the candidates as the possible sources for new ideas. The second step is to examine the relationship of the candidate biological models to various aspects of the technology problem at hand. The third step is to find the solution to the problem.

Among the whole design processes, this chapter covers the phases from "Development of ideas" to "Analogy/abstraction.", and OET has been developed for engineers as the main intended users but biologists should not be excluded.

2.2.3 An Envisioned Application

Concept formation is a key in the first phase of the design process. Before discussing our approach to it, we try to appeal to readers' intuition by giving a concrete example. We here present an application program we envision to demonstrate the potentials of OET. The application is named Keyword Explorer.

2.2.3.1 How Keyword Explorer works

Keyword Explorer is an application program running on OET to explore the space spanned by the concepts defined in OET considering each concept as a keyword for use of retrieval of relevant information. The exploration mechanism is association-based. See Fig. 2.2, in which rectangles denote concepts and links association (relation) defined in OET. When a user inputs antifouling, Keyword Explorer starts traverse of the keyword space spanned by OET like a person does association-based inference as follows:

> When it gets dirty, if it automatically cleans itself (self-cleaning), it would work for antifouling, to self-clean, washing out the dirt would be also effective. To do so, covering its surface with water would work well. Oh, it reminds me of hydrophilic property which in turn reminds me of water repellence. Roses are well-known as their hydrophilic property which is opposite to water repellence. Roses realize those two properties by their double structure which is shared also by lotus leaves. To find something antifouling, to investigate creatures living in the mud would be effective. Ummm, earthworms live in the mud and their surface look clean, etc., etc.

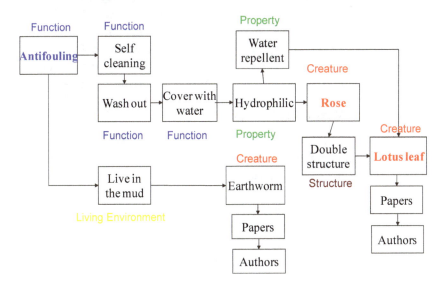

Figure 2.2 Association-based inference by Keyword explorer.

In such a way, users would be able to reach rose, lotus leaf, earthworm, etc. some of which would be useful to them. They can find papers about them and would be able to find more detailed information as well as experts on the related topics. What is important here from implementation perspectives is what knowledge has to be prepared for enabling such association-based inference. Let us investigate types of concepts appearing in the above example inference. Antifouling, self-cleaning, washing out and covering with water are functions, water repellent and hydrophilic are properties, rose, lotus leaf and earthworms are creatures and living in the mud is related to living environment. Furthermore, self-cleaning and washing out are sub-functions of antifouling function, and covering with water is a sub-function of self-cleaning, which suggests function-decomposition relation plays an important role to facilitate such an associative inference. We thus recognize the role played by ontologies in the knowledge infrastructure. See Fig. 2.1, which shows how the gap between engineering and biology are filled by these ontologies. Imagine, those two vertical ovals stand for conventional thesauri of engineering and biology domains, respectively. Although each thesaurus works well in the respective domain, they would be weak for biomimetics which is a composite of these two domains. This suggests that such ontologies can enhance the utility of conventional thesauri by bridging the gap between engineering and biology domains. This is how we conceptualize the notion of Ontology-Enhanced Thesaurus discussed in Section 2.5 in detail.

2.2.3.2 A Motivating Example

To consider a more concrete utility of Keyword Explorer, let us see the following example scenario. Imagine Jane, an engineer working in a house-construction company who is asked by her boss to invent a new eco-friendly idea for floors and walls. If she has little knowledge about tools of biomimetics, she will be in trouble and she has to work hard in reading many papers on success stories. But, when she notices a thesaurus could help her find better keywords for searching relevant papers, then she tries to find one. Assume she finds E2B thesaurus [40] developed based on the functional basis [29]. Her background is engineering, so what she comes up with in her mind include keywords such as "easy to clean" or "stain-resistant," so she expects E2B which translates between engineering and biological terms to be helpful. She tries to translate these two engineering terms, but fail to translate them into biological terms by E2B. In such a situation, she needs to somehow come up with appropriate technical terms used in databases as an index. Jane would be happier if she would receive a two-step help as follows:

The first step: Jane should find appropriate keywords that best capture her intention. At first, she only knows "stain-resistant" or "easy to clean", but with a help of a certain biomimetics thesaurus[1], she might be able to find "antifouling". When she types in "antifouling," biomimetics databases will return relevant information if it contains information about biological organisms that have antifouling properties. However, it is not realistic to expect all pieces of information potentially useful for her are successfully indexed by "antifouling." She will never notice such information that is not indexed by the term. Hence, there remains the issue of how to compensate for such missing links, in other words, how to fill the gap between her goal and the biological database with respect to "antifouling."

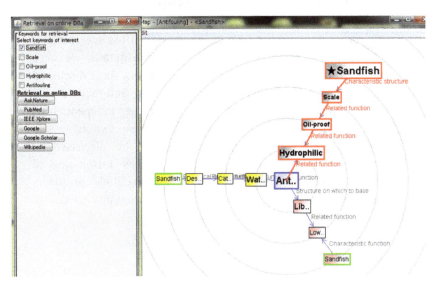

Figure 2.3 The case of sandfish and keywords found.

The second step (keyword exploration) might be able to help Jane to solve this issue using Keyword Explorer. It helps Jane find a set of appropriate keywords for her purpose by

---
[1] We do not assume any particular thesaurus here. It is not necessary because OET is loosely-coupled with a thesaurus. You could assume it would be what WG4 will produce in the near future.

allowing her to explore the keyword space spanned by the OET. Using Keyword Explorer, she might find organisms such as sandfish which is not directly indexed by "antifouling" function but somewhat related to it as well as well-known species such as lotus, snail, etc. Then she will be able to find information related to sandfish together with lotus and snail with additional keywords given by Keyword Explorer by collecting functions, features, etc. encountered during the association-based inference from "antifouling". Note here that, the second help provides only keywords for search as shown in Fig. 2.3. After that, users conduct detailed search using them to find relevant information from biomimetics databases such as Google, Google Scholar, AskNature, etc., as shown in the left pane in the figure.

2.3 Ontology-Enhanced Thesaurus

In this section, we discuss OET in the context of the specificity of the domain of biomimetics. Before going into details, we here clarify the relation between OET and a thesaurus. As is discussed in Section 2.2.3.2, OET and "thesaurus" is well-modularized or loosely coupled so that these two works rather independently. In other words, the interaction between these two is coarse enough to discuss them separately. It will be discussed in Section 2.3.3.1 in detail. A thesaurus solves terminological problems and OET solves so-called missing link problems discussed in Section 2.3.3.1. OET does not assume any particular thesaurus to enhance.

2.3.1 Characteristics of Biomimetics DBs

A biomimetics database is not an ordinary database which stores information about a single particular domain. It is an interdisciplinary database comprising not only databases of papers on biomimetics but also databases of all kinds of biological data, such as inventories, electron microscopy images, and experimental data. Therefore, interoperability of various kinds of data must be considered seriously.

According to such an interdisciplinary characteristic, differences between domains cause a couple of problems among which terminological difference is dominant. Engineers in biomimetics are not familiar with biological terms, and hence they do need substantial assistance in finding useful information about organisms that can be a source of creative ideas for developing innovative engineering products. The similar applies to biologists who are not familiar with engineering terms.

2.3.2 Basic Design of a Biomimetics Database Retrieval Scheme

Figure 2.4 shows an overview of future biomimetics databases with an advanced accompanying retrieval system which we envision on the basis of the above-mentioned characteristics and requirements. Various databases can be integrated by adding metadata to them based on the biomimetics ontology which should be implemented as Linked Open Data (LOD) to enable it to be linked to a variety of data on the Web. In addition, a sophisticated support system for retrieving information out of these interdisciplinary DBs would be available to exploit valuable data for innovative research.

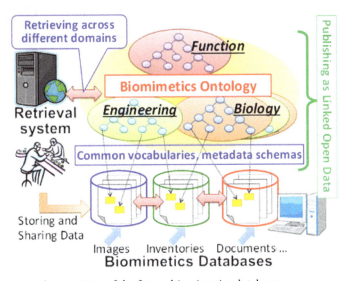

Figure 2.4 An overview of the future biomimetics databases.

Under the near future vision shown in Fig. 2.4, a future standard about this topic will produce a specification of development process of a concrete model of an advanced information retrieval system for biomimetics which we concretize as Ontology-Enhanced Thesaurus suggested in Section 2.2.3. We should note that we have no intention to build "The ontology of biomimetics". We are aware of the fact that it would be too early due to the immaturity of the domain. Rather, OET will cover mainly such ontologies that are specialized for bridging the gap between engineering and biology to make its activities manageable and feasible.

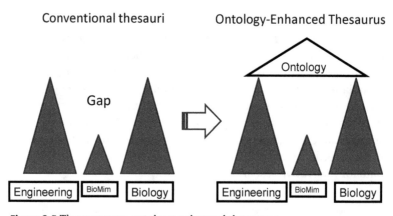

Figure 2.5 Thesaurus vs. ontology-enhanced thesaurus.

In general, users retrieving information from databases need to use appropriate keywords. Some retrieval systems provide users with a thesaurus, a systematic collection of related terms with their relationships, to help the users with that task. A thesaurus is built by exploiting documents about the target domain and its quality depends heavily on quantity and quality of the used documents. Unfortunately, biomimetics is a newly born research topic, and hence documents about it are not matured enough comparing with other matured domains (see the left in Fig. 2.5). Therefore, there is no guarantee that relations between terms used in the two domains (engineering and biology) are adequately covered by a thesaurus even if it is made for biomimetics. This is the reason why further enhancement would be required to augment the utility of biomimetics thesauri for bridging possible gaps between these two domains. OET is designed to realize such an augmented thesaurus for biomimetics (Fig. 2.5).

2.3.3 Keyword Exploration as an Independent Task before Issuing Queries to DBs

The example scenario presented in Section 2.2.3.2 shows how to help users find appropriate keywords to search for information across different domains. This is why we separate the tasks of finding keywords using Keyword Explorer from the main information retrieval tasks on the biomimetics database. Technically, the keyword finding task is implemented using a conventional thesaurus discussed in Section 2.4, and the keyword exploration is developed based on the ontology exploration tool [15, 16] using the biomimetics ontology. An important point here is that we divide cases where the keyword finding task is performed into two: a case where terminological difference matters and the other where missing links at the conceptual level matters. These cases are dealt with by keyword translation and exploration, respectively. The two methods are used not only sequentially but also simultaneously whenever they are needed. For instance, if a user finds an organism as a candidate for the target of a search, then he or she can use the help of the first step to solve a terminological problem before proceeding to the next search.

2.3.3.1 Keyword exploration and missing links

A concept appearing in a domain (e.g., engineering) does not always appear in others (e.g., biology). In such cases, even if some pieces of information which are indexed by a biological term denoting another concept deeply related to the engineering concept will not be found by engineers because there is no explicit link between these two concepts. We call such a case "missing link". Missing links between multiple domains should be compensated in order to allow engineers to find more useful information. In such cases, since no thesaurus can provide any help, we apply an ontology exploration tool [15, 16] which tries to contribute to bridging the gap caused by such missing links. A fundamental idea behind keyword exploration is to view those ontologies in OET as a network of abstract concepts linked by referencing relation between them.

Furthermore, if those ontologies are published as LOD, it would enable users to access other databases easily (e.g., just by clicking links). Large-scale LOD such as DBpedia[2] could be especially useful for acquiring an overview of a selected concept (keyword). Through such information obtained from other databases, users can find more important and appropriate keywords that they can use to search useful information stored in biomimetics databases.

2.3.3.2 Keyword exploration reasoning (divergent thinking and convergent thinking)

Keyword exploration for a biomimetics database aims to suggest users appropriate keywords to assist them in finding meaningful information for innovative biodiversity-based engineering. Note here that the proposed system gives users not the perfect solution for their requirements, but hints to stimulate idea creation. When we investigated the system architecture of Keyword Explorer, we had two choices: a carefully tailored heuristic search and a generic inference engine. After some discussion, we finally decided to adopt the latter for decreasing the domain-specificity of the application. We then faced the next issue of selecting an inference engine. Since its main purpose is stimulating idea creation, keyword exploration does not require an engine based on strict reasoning because it would show only inferable knowledge that users can expect by logical reasoning, whereas what they need is a help for finding unexpected data/information for idea creation. That is, rough inference is more suitable for idea creation than strict reasoning, since it simulates so-called **divergent thinking** even though its results could include useless or rubbish information. Of course, users must investigate the results of such help to confirm their utility. An ontology exploration tool developed on top of OET supports such a rough inference by employing association-based inference explained in Section 2.2.3.1 and helps users find unexpected relationships

---

[2]http://dbpedia.org/.

among concepts [7]. For the same reason, the ontology in OET covers broader concepts without much detailed definition when it is used for keyword exploration.

In addition to the divergent thinking based on the association-based inference, Keyword Explorer provides users with **convergent thinking** to allow them to narrow down the candidate information. After suggesting candidate organisms to explore, it can show users a set of relevant keywords by collecting all the concepts on the paths to the user-selected organisms obtained by the associate-based inference as shown in the left pane of Fig. 2.3. By combining appropriate concepts as keywords, users easily retrieve relevant information on several DBs available on-line, which drastically speeds up their information search. Keyword Explorer thus facilitates both divergent and convergent thinking processes of users based on the ontology built in OET.

2.3.3.3 Two-step help

To resolve terminological differences in different domains, we first introduce conventional thesaurus built from available resources in biomimetics. We believe it works well but its effect would be limited due to specificity of biomimetics discussed earlier. In order to make up for such possible inefficiency, we introduce an additional task of "keyword exploration" before performing actual information retrieval. Finding an appropriate set of keywords is critical to a success of finding useful information in DBs. In cases where keywords provided by a biomimetics thesaurus are not satisfactory, users need additional help to find better keywords. This is why we find a necessity to enhance capacity of biomimetics thesauri. OET plays an important role in the keyword exploration task. In fact, abstract concepts defined in the ontology in OET provide a useful common vocabulary for associative inference. Through dynamic linking of terms in the thesaurus and concepts in the ontology, an ordinary thesaurus is enhanced to extend its capability of relating seemingly different terms. Technically, we offer two-step mediation discussed in Section 2.2.3.2 using the ontology according to two possible situations where users need effective support such as (1) A same concept appears in multiple domains but they are terminologically different and (2) A pair of concepts denoted by different terms are semantically related to each other but there are no explicit passes (links) between them (missing link).

2.4 Ontologies in OET

We have discussed the design philosophy of OET and the two-step keyword search on OET in the context of the envisioned biomimetics databases in the last section. In this section, we discuss what ontologies we have developed to exemplify a prototype of OET.

2.4.1 Basic Design of Ontologies in OET

According to a preliminary study about how engineers use biomimetics database and the example presented in Section 2.3, we envisioned the basic design of the biomimetics ontology as shown in Fig. 2.6. OET is composed of a couple of ontologies on top of a thesaurus built for biomimetics by a conventional way. In fact, most successful examples are model-based imitations of capabilities that organisms possess, such as the water repellency of a lotus and the adhesiveness of gecko's feet. We considered that a key concept in compensating for the missing links is the relationship between the target function and such creatures that already realized it. Its living environment is another key concept because it is closely related to typical behaviors/features.

2.4.2 Ontology of Function

OET and Keyword Explorer rely on the ontology of function [18]. In spite of the importance of the ontology of function, however, its details are omitted due to the strong theoretical characteristics.

2.4.3 Concepts other than Function

A unique feature of the biomimetics ontologies in OET is that not only they are right ontologies by themselves but also they are designed for Keyword Explorer to explore the keyword space and to effectively make up for "missing links". In other words, the latter requires them of a characteristic of divergent exploration by which we mean association-based trace of all links to related concepts [39]. This will lead users to find unexpected but useful information. In addition to functional ontology, biomimetics ontology we have implemented in OET includes ontology of a taxonomy of creatures, properties, and living environments as discussed below.

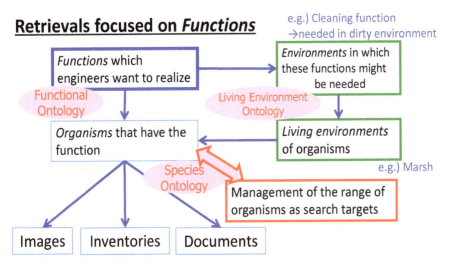

Figure 2.6 Components of the biomimetics ontology and how they are used to retrieve biomimetics databases.

2.4.3.1 Taxonomy of creatures

The target of keyword exploration is creatures which might have relevant functions/structures for engineers. The most serious issue we face here would be the fact that there exist a large number of creatures on the earth so that it is impossible to store all of them with reasonable amount of property descriptions in an ontology. Therefore, we adopted a realistic strategy on this matter. We first stored most of the known creatures appearing in every success story we have to date. Many of the creatures similar to them are also collected. The most apparent strategy, however, would be to collect candidates from biologists who are experts of quite a few kinds of creatures. So, we asked colleagues working together in the Japanese project on biomimetics for typical creatures they know with description about its properties, functions, typical behaviors, anatomical structure and living environments. The total number of creatures in the current OET is about 350.

2.4.3.2 Properties

Description of creatures requires an ontology of properties such as weight, size, temperature, color, etc. Terminology about property is a mess. So, we need a good ontological foundation about properties to deal with them appropriately. There are several similar terms such as attribute, characteristic, property, quality, quantity, attribute value, etc. Imagine someone claims "height is a property" and another "tall is a property" Apparently these two are incompatible because only one of the two is correct. We have to have a correct answer to each of them and to have a firm justification to the decision together with the answer of what a property is. If we believe tall is a property, then we have to answer why it is not an attribute value. Many of OWL people believe a property is a relation between an object and property (attribute) value. But it is wrong ontologically. A property is not a relation but a dependent entity.

Although there exist two well-established upper ontologies such as DOLCE [20] and BFO [21], neither can settle down those issues. So, we adopted YAMATO [22] as an example of upper ontology which is the only upper ontology which can settle down such fundamental issues related to properties.

2.4.3.3 Living environments

Although its utility is rather indirect, this item is very important. Ontology of living environments is selected because it is used for suggesting that creatures which live in a particular environment might have a particular function to cope with or enjoy the particular characteristic of the environment. The utility was already suggested by the earthworm example in Section 2.2.3.1. Each living environment is also described in terms of properties which characterize its peculiarity such as a desert is dry and hot.

2.4.3.4   The quality of ontologies in OET

There are two kinds of qualities about biomimetics ontology: One is (a) quality from the ontological/theoretical perspectives and the other is (b) quality from domain-dependent content perspectives. Frankly speaking, however, the requirement for quality from either perspective is not very demanding in OET. It can be rough instead, since the inference performed on the biomimetics ontology is based on association rather than a rigid logical inference. As a minimum requirement of the coverage which is one of the qualities from content perspectives, we at least chose all the terms used in all the documents of other international standards and those in most of the successful stories.

2.5   Implementation and Evaluation of a Prototype of Keyword Explorer

Keyword Explorer has been implemented on top of the prototype OET and it is ready for the evaluation to get feedback from users. The implementation has been done intended to cover only the second-step help discussed in Sections 2.2.3.2 and 2.3.3.3 because the first-step help is not innovative and those two kinds of help are independent from each other (Fig. 2.7) [15, 16].

Two versions of Keyword Explorer have been implemented. One is just a demo system and the other is a prototype version which runs on a prototype OET. The demo version is a lightweight version intended to let possible users to capture how Keyword Explorer works and to get motivated to use the prototype version.

2.5.1   Implementation of Keyword Explorer

The fundamental functionality of these two implemented systems is essentially the same. The demo version is a Web application which accesses the ontology of OET of the demo version and the prototype version works as a local application after the download. The major difference is the size of the ontology.

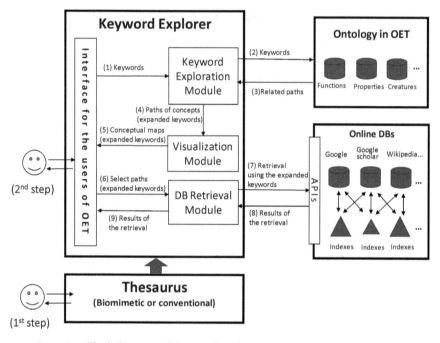

Figure 2.7 Block diagram of Keyword explorer.

2.5.1.1 The demo version

The demo version is available at the demo site[3]. The corresponding ontology can be **browsed** on the site, though its download is not allowed.

2.5.1.2 The prototype version

Keyword Explorer of the prototype version runs on the local computers with the ontology of the prototype OET. Although the download of the prototype OET is not available because of an organizational reason, its use cases are found at the demo site for OET.

The prototype OET provides four kinds of engineering functions such as:

(1) Antifouling
(2) Low friction

---

[3]http://biomimetics.hozo.jp/OET/.

(3) Adhesion

(4) Sensing

That is, users can start either one of these four functions for exploration of all possible paths to candidate creatures in the search space spanned by about 350 species implemented with their properties, structures, behaviors and functions together with function decompositions of important functions

2.5.2   Preliminary Evaluation Experiment

A preliminary experiment has been done in Japan. We asked 20 companies belonging to a Special Interest Group (SIG) on Biomimetics in Japan to evaluate the utility of Keyword Explorer according to the following procedure:

Step 1: After a brief introduction and a demo of the Keyword Explorer, they were given two weeks for trial use.

Step 2: The Java-implemented tool was downloaded from a site in Osaka University.

Step 3: The ontology is hidden to the users and the tool runs accessing the ontology server at Osaka University.

Step 4: We asked them to return answers to a prepared questionnaire and 14 answers were returned out of 20 after two weeks.

Most of the members of the SIG are beginners of biomimetics/ BID and are looking for new research targets. As far as we understand, however, beginner or expert is not the critical factor in the talk about the utility of Keyword Explorer. This is because engineers in the phase of finding new research topics necessarily need such help that Keyword Explorer provides to find possible candidate organisms, since they lack biological knowledge anyway.

The result was encouraging. Five of them answered "very promising" and six "promising" to the question "Do you think this tool can help you find useful hints for innovative design of materials/devices?" The answers of "neutral" were only three. In addition, all answered "yes" to the question "Do you want to use this tool after revision and enhancement?" As to the functionality of the tool, although some room for future improvement was suggested by some of the users, majority of them were satisfied with the current functions of the prototype. Two among 14 said they were almost ready to write a new proposal of future development plan thanks to the useful information they got by this trial use. In summary, Keyword Explorer running on the current implementation of OET works satisfactorily for engineers working in biomimetics who look for new ideas.

2.6 Concluding Remarks

We understand Keyword Explorer and OET are rather new ideas and not widely spread in the world yet despite that the potential usefulness of Keyword Explorer in practice. This section discusses several issues about how OET can contribute to completion of the mission of TC266 and shows there are good reasons for future standardization of the development process of OET when Keyword Explorer and OET has become matured enough.

(1) Needs of knowledge infrastructure: Let us first briefly review the needs of engineers working in biomimetics. There can be two kinds of needs: one is at the engineering perspective and the other is scientific perspective. At the first perspective, while engineers who are in charge of BID badly need relevant information about candidate organisms/creatures for innovative products, conventional thesauri are not powerful enough because of the immaturity of the biomimetics. At the scientific perspective, on the other hand, the domain of biomimetics needs not only standard of terminology/vocabulary but also knowledge infrastructure to make its status more solid. The knowledge infrastructure serves as the foundation of the domain of biomimetics on top of which new findings and knowledge are built and organized to enable accumulation of scientific achievements for future computer-supported design activities following BID methodology.

(2) Beyond terminology: The terminology/vocabulary and characteristic processes of biomimetics have been standardized in WG1 and WG2 of TC266 to contribute to clarification of the notion of biomimetics. Although it is valuable to define biomimetics, we can go further to complete the goal by extending and enhancing those achievements to knowledge infrastructure and by covering the first phase of engineering process and enabling mutual understanding between engineers and biologists.

(3) An issue of ontology building: An ontology is expected to be a candidate of knowledge infrastructure. An issue, however, is there is no common or usable guideline for development of a good and useful ontology. It is partly because of the nature of an ontology. A theoretically good ontology has to be generic to cover wide range of domain concepts and hence tends to be weak in practice, whereas an application-oriented ontology developed for solving a particular type of problems has little generality and hence it cannot serve as a knowledge infrastructure of the domain. This observation suggests we need a convincing method for building such an ontology that can provide practical benefits while keeping its strength as a knowledge infrastructure of the biomimetics domain. OET and its development process are expected to resolve such conflicting requirements.

References

1. Hirtz J., Stone R. B., et Al. (2002). A functional basis for engineering design: reconciling and evolving previous effort, NIST Technical Note 1447.

2. Kitamura Y., Segawa S., Sasajima M., Tarumi S., Mizoguchi R. (2008). Deep semantic mapping between functional taxonomies for interoperable semantic search, *Proceeding of the 3rd Asian Semantic Web Conference (ASWC 2008)*, LNCS 5367, February 2–5, Bangkok, Thailand, pp. 137–151.

3. Scherge M., Gorb, S. (2001). *Biological Micro- and Nanotribology.* Springer-Verlag, ISBN 3-540-41188-7.

4. Forbes P. (2005). *The Gecko's Foot: Bio-inspiration: Engineering New Materials and Devices from Nature.* Fourth Estate Ltd., August 15, 2005, ISBN 0007179901, 288 pages, hardcover.

5. Gruber P. (2011). *Biomimetics in Architecture: Architecture of Life and Buildings*, 1st ed, 280 p. 466 illus., Softcover, ISBN: 978-3-7091-0331-9.

6. Webb B (ed). (2001). Consi, Thomas R. *Biorobotics, Methods & Applications.* AAAI Press/The MIT Press, London, ISBN: 026273141X, 250 pages.

7. Iida F. Pfeifer R. Steels L. *Embodied Artificial Intelligence,* Springer, Berlin, Jul 2004, ISBN: 354022484X, 330 pages.

8. Mattheck C., Kubler H. (1997). *Wood: The Internal Optimization of Trees,* Springer Verlag, Heidelberg, 2. Auflage.

9. Mattheck C., Breloer H. (1996). *The Body Language of Trees: A Handbook for Failure Analysis HMSO,* London, 2. Auflage.

10. *Bioinspiration & Biomimetics.* http://iopscience.iop.org/1748-3190.

11. *International Journal of Design & Nature and Ecodynamics.* http://journals.witpress.com/jdne.asp.

12. George A. *Advances in Biomimetics.* InTech, April 26, 2011, ISBN 978-953-307-191-6, 532 pages.

13. Goel A. K., McAdams D. A., Stone R. B. (2014). *Biologically Inspired Design: Computational Methods and Tools.* Springer, England.

14. Cheong H., Chiu I., Shu L. H., Stone R. B., McAdams D. A. (2011). Biologically meaningful keywords for functional terms of the functional basis. *Journal of Mechanical Design,* **133**(2), 021007.

15. Kozaki K., Hirota T., Mizoguchi R. (2011). Understanding an ontology through divergent exploration. *Proceedings of ESWC 2011,* Part I, LNCS 6643, pp. 305–320.

16. Kouji K., Riichiro M. (2014). A keyword exploration for retrieval from biomimetics databases, *Proceedings of JIST2014.*

17. Kitamura Y., Mizoguchi R. (2003). Ontology-based description of functional design knowledge and its use in a functional way server. *Expert Systems with Applications,* **24**(2), 153–166.

18. Kitamura Y., Segawa S., Sasajima M., Tarumi S., Mizoguchi R. (2008). Deep semantic mapping between functional taxonomies for interoperable semantic search, *Proceedings of the 3rd Asian Semantic Web Conference (ASWC 2008),* LNCS 5367, pp. 137–151, February 2–5, Bangkok, Thailand.

19. Mizoguchi R. (2004). Tutorial on ontological engineering: Parts 1, 2, 3. *New Generation Computing,* **22**(2), 193–220.

20. http://www.loa.istc.cnr.it/old/DOLCE.html.

21. http://ifomis.uni-saarland.de/bfo/.

22. http://download.hozo.jp/onto_library/upperOnto.htm.

23. https://asknature.org/.

24. http://www.biotriz.com/our-methods.

25. http://shulab.mie.utoronto.ca/ (BIDLab).

26. Vincent J. F. V., Bogatyreva O. A., Bogatyrev N. R., Bowyer A., Pahl A.-K. (2006). Biomimetics: its practice and theory. *Journal of the Royal Society Interface*, **3**(9), 471–482.

27. Bogatyrev N., Bogatyreva O. (2014). BioTRIZ: a win-win methodology for eco-innovation, in *Eco-innovation and the Development of Business Models: Lessons from Experience and New Frontiers in Theory and Practice*, Springer, pp. 297–314.

28. Chakrabarti A., Sarkar P., Leelavathamma B., Nataraju B. (2005). A functional representation for aiding biomimetic and artificial inspiration of new ideas. *Artificial Intelligence for Engineering Design, Analysis and Manufacturing*, **19**(2), 113–132.

29. Shu L. H., Stone R. B., McAdams D. A., Greer J. L. (2007). *Integrating Function-Based and Biomimetic Design for Automatic Concept Generation*, International Conference on Engineering Design (ICED'07), Paris, France, August 28–31.

30. Vattam S., Helms M., Goel A. (2009). *Nature of Creative Analogies in Biologically Inspired Innovative Design*, C&C Proceedings of the Seventh ACM Conference on Creativity and Cognition, New York, pp. 255–264.

31. Jacobs S. R., Nichol E. C., Helms M. E. (2014). "Where are we now and where are we going?" The BioM innovation database. *Journal of Mechanical Design*, 136, 111101 1–10.

32. Markus H. H. (2012). *Hollermann: Enabling Biomimetics—Development and Evaluation of a Biomimetic Methodology for Supporting Creativity in Product Innovation*, Master Thesis, University of Bremen, August 1.

33. http://www.obofoundry.org/.

34. https://en.wikipedia.org/wiki/Ontology_(information_science).

35. https://en.wikipedia.org/wiki/Metadata.

36. https://en.wikipedia.org/wiki/TRIZ.

37. Nagel J. K. S., Stone R. B., McAdams D. A. (2010). *An Engineering-to-Biology: Thesaurus for Engineering Design*, Proceedings of the ASME 2010 International Design Engineering Technical Conferences & Computers and Information in Engineering Conference IDETC/CIE 2010, August 15–18, 2010, Montreal, Quebec, Canada, 1–11, 2010.

38. http://bioinspired.sinet.ca/content/biom-innovation-database.

39. Kumazawa T., Saito O., Kozaki K., Matsui T., Mizoguchi R. (2009). Toward knowledge structuring of sustainability science based on ontology engineering. *Sustainability Science*, **4**(1), 99–116.

40. file:///C:/Users/miz/Downloads/E2BThesaurusv2.pdf.

41. http://dilab.cc.gatech.edu/dane/.

42. Chiu I., Shu L. H. (2007). Biomimetic design through natural-language analysis to facilitate cross-domain information retrieval. AIEDAM **21**(1), 45–59.

43. Cheong H., Chiu I., Shu L. H., Stone R., McAdams D. (2011). Biologically meaningful keywords for functional terms of the functional basis. *ASME The Journal of Mechanical Design*, **133**, 021007.

44. Vincent J. F. V. (2016). The trade-off: a central concept for biomimetics. *Bioinspired, Biomimetic and Nanobiomaterials*, **6**(2), 67–76.

Chapter 3

Biomimetics Image Retrieval Platform for Bridging Different Study Fields

Miki Haseyama and Takahiro Ogawa

Faculty of Information Science and Technology,
Hokkaido University, N-14, W-9, Kita-ku
Sapporo, Hokkaido060-0814, Japan

miki@ist.hokudai.ac.jp, ogawa@lmd.ist.hokudai.ac.jp

Biomimetics is a new field in which innovations are achieved by strong collaboration between different existing study fields. By exchanging knowledge between different study fields, the development of new technologies becomes feasible. However, since collaboration between different study fields is difficult, it is an obstacle for developing new technologies. For example, since technical terms (terminologies) in different study fields are different, exchange of knowledge is difficult. In order to solve this problem, we have proposed a new image retrieval platform called "biomimetics image retrieval platform" for finding commonness between image data obtained from different study fields. In the field of biology, many scanning electron microscope (SEM) images have been taken, and our platform can determine similarities between these SEM images and images

---

Biomimetics: Connecting Ecology and Engineering by Informatics
Edited by Akihiro Miyauchi and Masatsugu Shimomura
Copyright © 2023 Jenny Stanford Publishing Pte. Ltd.
ISBN 978-981-4968-10-2 (Hardcover), 978-1-003-27717-0 (eBook)
www.jennystanford.com

in other study fields such as material science. By focusing on the visual characteristics of images, the above-mentioned problem can be solved since we do not have to consider the difference between the technical terms. Consequently, our biomimetics image retrieval platform provides users with a new path for bridging different study fields to contribute to the development of new technologies in biomimetics.

3.1 Introduction

Biomimetics has become well known as a new study field yielding novel manufacturing concepts on the basis of structures, functionality and reproduction processes of natural organisms [1, 2]. It has recently attracted much attention since it has high potential for realizing a sustainable society. Many new engineering technologies have been developed by focusing on unique characteristics of natural organisms. By artificially reproducing nanostructures (surfaces) of bio-organisms having useful characteristics, i.e., unique functions, a number of nanomaterials have been developed. Unique engineering developments can be realized by collaboration between different existing study fields such as biology and material science fields.

Since studies in biomimetics are carried out by collaboration between at least two different study fields for which there had been no collaboration in the past, close collaboration is mandatory. Furthermore, since biomimetics is based on the study of biology, researchers in engineering fields need to have biological knowledge. However, obtaining such knowledge is difficult due to the large biodiversity, i.e., it is difficult to find new characteristics among many kinds of biological organisms. Even if engineering researchers know target characteristics, it is still difficult to find the corresponding biological organisms due to the differences of technical terms (terminologies).

Recently, various improvements have been made to SEMs. SEM images are now often taken in various study fields. For example, researchers in biology use SEMs for observing subcellular structures on surfaces of various kinds of bio-organisms. Researchers in the fields of nanomaterials and nanofabrication also take SEM images for observing structures. In biomimetics, engineering researchers can find unique structures of biological organisms from SEM images and can reproduce them to realize desired functions in materials. In order to strengthen this approach, it is necessary for engineering researchers to be able to access various SEM image data in biological fields, which are separately accumulated for various kinds of biological organisms, and find their corresponding biological researchers.

In order to satisfy the above necessity, we have to focus on the following two points: (1) integration of SEM images separately accumulated in various biological study fields and (2) development of a novel image retrieval platform. For (1), the cooperation of museums that have accumulated samples and their corresponding information related to this vast diversity would provide an effective solution. Museums play an important role in the accumulation of the information and provide seeds for biomimetics. However, an image retrieval platform for finding common structures in different study fields has not been considered. SEM images of common structures in different study fields have similar visual characteristics even if their terminology for describing certain properties is completely different. Therefore, it would be possible to retrieve these image data based on visual similarities.

In order to satisfy the above demand, we have developed a novel image retrieval platform called "biomimetics image retrieval platform" in which a visualization-based image retrieval technique is used [3]. The proposed platform uses similarities of visual features in SEM images to visualize all of the image data accumulated by biological researchers in a lower-dimensional space that is viewable by users. If nanostructures in two SEM images are similar, these images are placed at positions close to each other in the visualization space. This characteristic holds for images in both the same study field and different study fields since visual characteristics are not affected by differences in terminologies. Therefore, by using the proposed platform, engineering researchers can find SEM images that include similar nanostructures from different fields such as biology to discover new inter-field collaborations. This means that our platform provides researchers with new paths potentially existing between different study fields. Consequently, new developments in biomimetics can be expected since our platform drastically breaks the limitations of existing retrieval engines.

3.2 Background for New Image Retrieval Platform

3.2.1 Need for an Image Retrieval Scheme in Biomimetics Studies

As shown in the introduction, researchers in biomimetics belong to different study fields and try to generate innovation via their collaborations. Although they need to exchange their own specific knowledge with each other, understanding different study fields is difficult since their terminologies are different. Such differences cause obstacles for the exchange of knowledge, and mutual understandings in different fields also become difficult. Inter-field construction of dictionaries and ontologies is one solution for overcoming such obstacles, and its effectiveness in the field of biomimetics has been verified [4].

We focus on another solution using a unique characteristic observed in SEM images and try to create breakthroughs for overcoming the problem of such obstacles. Even if terminologies are different in different study fields, SEM images taken in their fields have similar visual characteristics when they have common nanostructures. Therefore, by comparing visual features obtained from SEM images and visualizing their relationships, we can find the common structures among different study fields.

3.2.2 Image Retrieval Based on a Visualization Technique

Many image retrieval engines have been developed in recent years. The existing retrieval engines are based on metadata, such as text, attached to image contents. Traditionally, these metadata have been attached manually or based on surrounding texts. On the other hand, with the rapid growth of multimedia data analysis, i.e., their semantic understanding, automatic estimation of such metadata has become feasible. Metadata can now be automatically attached to image and video contents. Recently, since deep learning technologies have attracted attention worldwide [5], the performance of these technologies for general object recognition has been greatly improved [6]. Although the image and video understanding performance becomes enough for general image recognition tasks, it is still difficult to realize the same performance for images taken in specific fields, i.e., images accumulated in the above-mentioned research fields, due to the lack of data for training. Furthermore, it would be impossible to prepare a sufficient amount of training data in the field of biomimetics. Although many images have been taken for various bio-organisms, the number of images taken for each species is still small. Furthermore, when focusing on SEM images, the above problem becomes much more significant since only a few images are taken for each part of each bio-organism at each magnification.

We also have to consider another problem that has recently become significant. We sometimes cannot provide suitable query keywords representing our desired images, and it is difficult to obtain desired images by using the existing retrieval engines [7–9]. A new retrieval platform needs to be developed to overcome this problem. It should be noted that in the field of biomimetics, this point becomes more important. As mentioned above, since terminologies are different in different study fields, it is difficult for engineering researchers to provide suitable queries.

As shown in the above explanation, it is difficult for existing retrieval engines to realize successful retrieval for providing new discoveries. In order to solve this problem, we have proposed a new retrieval approach that uses visualization schemes for providing users' desired images from a huge image database [10–13]. Our retrieval approach visualizes all of the images included in an image database according to their similarities, and users can easily understand their relationships in the database. Users do not have to prepare suitable queries and can successfully find their desired images.

Our previously proposed image retrieval engines target not only image data but also various unstructured data, and realize their visualization. Specifically, numerical features are calculated from target unstructured data, and these data are visualized in low-dimensional spaces (equal to or less than three-dimensional spaces) according to the similarities of the calculated features. The first prototype of our visualization-based retrieval engines is "Image Vortex" [11] shown in Fig. 3.1. This image retrieval engine was developed to provide a solution to the problem of traditional retrieval engines not being able to achieve successful retrieval when users cannot provide suitable queries. This retrieval engine calculates visual features from images in the target database and defines distances between the visual features [14, 15]. Then, on the basis of the obtained distances, the images in the target database are visualized in a three-dimensional space obtained by a dimensionality reduction scheme as shown in Fig. 3.1. From the interface shown in this figure, we can see an overview of the target database, e.g., distributions of images and relationships between images, and we can easily find our desired images.

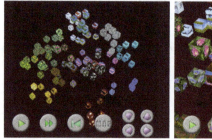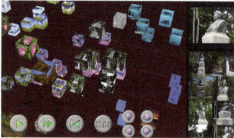

Figure 3.1 The visualization-based image retrieval engine "Image Vortex." This retrieval engine enables users to find relationships between images in the target database based on similarities of their visual features.

By extending Image Vortex to a much larger-scale database, we have developed a new cloud-based image retrieval engine called "Image Cruiser" (Fig. 3.2). Compared to Image Vortex, Image Cruiser has enhanced "scalability" (increase in the number of images in the target database) and greater "computation speed" (fast retrieval) for realizing a cloud-based retrieval platform. By introducing the interface shown in Fig. 3.2, users can find an overview of the database and successfully reach their desired images. As for Image Vortex, Image Cruiser does not need any queries, i.e., query images/texts, from users.

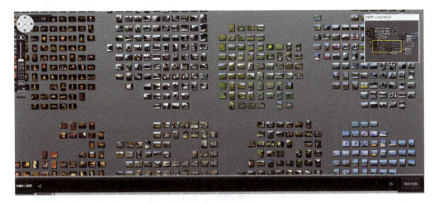

Figure 3.2 The large-scale image retrieval engine "Image Cruiser." This cloud-based retrieval engine has enhanced scalability and computation speed for realizing visualization of a large amount of image data.

3.3 Biomimetics Image Retrieval Platform

3.3.1 Algorithm in Our Retrieval Platform

First, we explain the algorithm used in our novel image retrieval platform; biomimetics image retrieval platform. Our platform is based on the concept of visualization-based image retrieval explained in the previous section. The platform visualizes the whole database including SEM images to enable users to understand its overview. This can be realized by dimensionality reduction of visual features to a two-dimensional visualization space. This dimensionality reduction-based visualization is realized by the algorithm shown in [11]. By using a two-dimensional visualization interface, it is possible for users to understand an overview of the target SEM image database and find their desired SEM images.

The algorithm of the biomimetics image retrieval platform is composed of the following three steps.

Step 1. Visual feature calculation from SEM images

Several visual features are extracted from SEM images. Specifically, features based on color histograms and correlograms obtained from the whole image and its target object are calculated. Principal component analysis is applied to the extracted visual features to reduce their dimensions. In recent years, better visual features have been proposed with the growth of deep learning technologies, and it will be useful to introduce such features.

Step 2. Distance calculation of dimensionality-reduced visual features

The distances of the dimensionality-reduced visual features obtained in Step 1 are calculated for all of the pairs of SEM images in the database. In this image retrieval platform, the Euclidean distance is used for this step. More suitable distances may be selected for a target image database, and distance metric learning will lead to improvement of the following retrieval performance.

Step 3. Visualization of SEM images in two-dimensional space

The image platform introduces a dimensionality reduction algorithm [11] to the distances calculated in the previous step for determining the positions in the two-dimensional visualization space. The dimensionality reduction algorithm can be replaced by recently proposed methods.

As shown in each step, the algorithms for feature extraction, distance calculation and dimensionality reduction can be replaced by more suitable algorithms for the target image database. With the growth of the deep learning technologies, each algorithm has been improved by introducing deep structures. Therefore, our image retrieval platform has a high degree of freedom. Note that since SEM images accumulated in the biomimetics image retrieval platform tend to include only simple textures, we use the simple algorithms shown in the above steps for low-computational complexity.

3.3.2 Functions Equipped in the Biomimetics Image Retrieval Platform

The background algorithm in the biomimetics image retrieval platform was explained in the previous subsection. In this subsection, the main functions equipped in the retrieval platform are explained. Specifically, this platform provides visualization-based image retrieval of SEM images in the study field of biology, and users can find suitable SEM images that are useful for engineering.

(A) Overview visualization of the target SEM image database

An overview of the whole SEM image database is visualized as shown in Fig. 3.3. In this figure, some important items are included as functions of the visualization interface, and their details are shown below. First, an overview of the whole image database is shown in Fig. 3.3(a). By changing settings by the function in Fig. 3.3(b), the number and size of the visualized images can be changed. Users can watch and find their desired images from this interface, and the bottom region shown in Fig. 3.3(c) provides the viewing history of the target user.

(B) Bio-organism information confirmation

After finding the desired SEM images from the target database, users need to confirm their detailed information. Therefore, the biomimetics image retrieval platform provides details, inventory information, of selected bio-organisms as shown in Fig. 3.4. Representative information is shown in Table 3.1. By selecting useful inventory information, new retrieval using the selected information becomes feasible by narrowing down the visualized images. An example obtained by using this function is shown in Fig. 3.5. By limiting the retrieved targets from the inventory information, the visualized SEM images can be narrowed down. The example shows the results obtained by limiting the magnification of SEM images. When engineering researchers use this retrieval interface and can find their desired nanostructures from bio-organisms, they can obtain important information. In the inventory information, some useful keywords are included. Eco. Keywords are representative ones, which include important information for biomimetics and are unique items in our platform, such as moth-eye, anti-reflectivity, hydrophobic, structural adhesion, structural color, photonic crystal, etc.

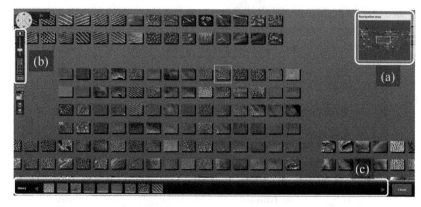

Figure 3.3 The visualization interface of the biomimetics image retrieval platform. Users can understand the overview of the image database in (a). By using the function in (b), users can change the number and size of visualized images. The viewing history is also shown in (c).

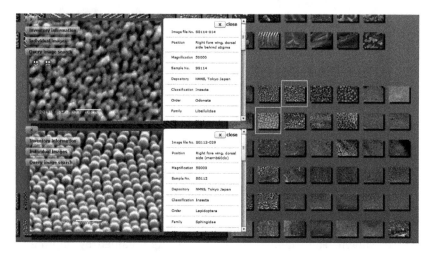

Figure 3.4 Display of inventory information (bio-organism information) of selected SEM images.

Table 3.1 Representative inventory information provided by the biomimetics image retrieval platform. The information is attached to each bio-organism image

Order	Magnification	Position	Genus	Depository
Classification	Sex	Family	JPN name	Collector
Species	Subspecies	Eco. Keywords	Locality	Method
Coating	Habitat	Camera	Photographer	Size (mm)

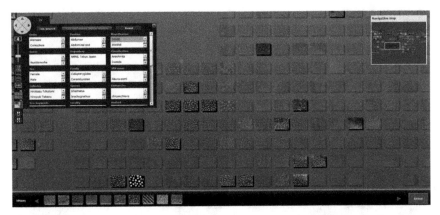

Figure 3.5 Function for narrowing down the visualized images. In this example, only images with magnification of ×30000 are selected, and other images are grayed out.

(C) Retrieval from query keywords

As stated in (B), each SEM image has inventory information in the biomimetics image retrieval platform. Therefore, if the target user knows specific inventory information about the desired bio-organisms, our retrieval platform can provide keyword query-based retrieval. An example of results obtained by query keyword-based retrieval is shown in Fig. 3.6. It should be noted that as stated in the previous section, retrieval based on keywords is generally difficult due to the differences of terminologies in different study fields, e.g., biology and material science. Furthermore, as also stated in the previous section, dictionary and ontology construction for connecting different technical terms in different study fields is effective for overcoming the problem of the gap caused in keyword-based image retrieval. Furthermore, by adopting keywords such as Eco. Keywords that can be commonly used in different fields, our image retrieval platform provides new paths for engineering researchers to find their desired information, i.e., SEM images and their unique nanostructures.

(D) Retrieval from query images

The biomimetics image retrieval platform includes a function of query image retrieval. As shown in Fig. 3.7,

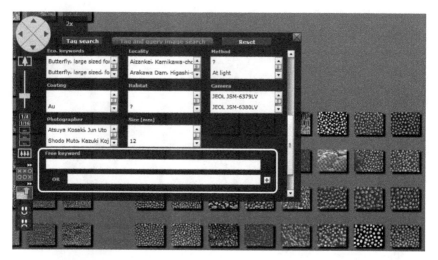

Figure 3.6 Function for keyword-based retrieval. From keywords input by users, images including these keywords can be selected.

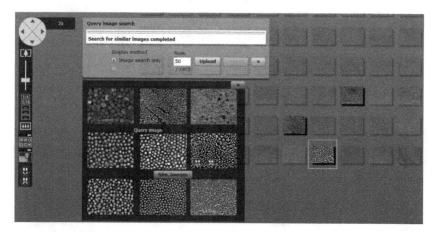

Figure 3.7 Function for image retrieval from a query image uploaded by users. The query image is shown at the center of the window, and eight similar images, i.e., the retrieval results, surrounding the query image are shown.

the eight images surrounding the query image arethe retrieved SEM images that includesimilar visual structures. This function is not affected by the difference of terminologies. Therefore, engineering researchers can find suitable bio-organisms that includesimilarnanostructures from the target biological database.

3.3.3 Inter-field Similarities Discovered by Our Platform

We show an inter-field similarity discovered by using the biomimetics image retrieval platform, where these results have reported in [3]. As shown in Figs. 3.8 and 3.9, we consider the case of a material scientist uploading four material SEM images and trying to find images of bio-organisms. The retrieval results shown in Figs. 3.8 and 3.9 were obtained. In the lower area of Fig. 3.8, there exist the following images.

- SEM images of the micro lens array produced based on [16]
- SEM image of the moth-eye structure of *Helicoverpa armigera*
- SEM image of the wings of the cicada *Terpnosia nigricosta*
- SEM image of the surface of the front wings of *Graptopsaltria bimaculata*

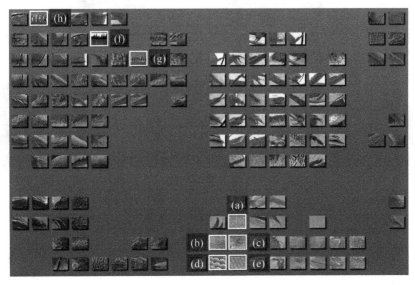

Figure 3.8 Examples obtained by the biomimetics image retrieval platform. The details of similar images in (a)–(e) and those in (f)–(h) are shown in Fig. 3.9.

The SEM images of *Helicoverpa armigera* and *Terpnosia nigricosta* were provided by Dr. Takahiko Hariyama in Hamamatsu University School of Medicine, and the other SEM images of insects were provided by Dr. Shuhei Nomura in National Museum of Nature. As shown in Figs. 3.8 and 3.9, SEM images of the silicon nanospike array produced based on [16] in the field of material science are placed closely to those of the wing cross-section of *Terpnosia nigricosta*. From the retrieval results shown in these figures, we can see that visual features obtained from similar surface structures can provide useful retrieval results even if their fields are different (i.e., biology and material science).

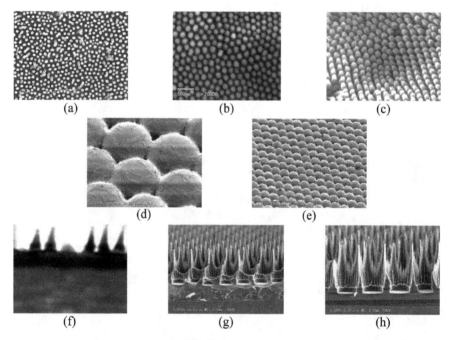

Figure 3.9 Images selected in Fig. 3.8: (a) Helicoverpa armigera (Noctuidae), (b) Terpnosia nigricosta (Cicadidae), (c) Graptopsaltria bimaculata (Cicadidae), (d) and (e) micro lens array (material images), (f) Terpnosia nigricosta (Cicadidae), and (g) and (h) silicon nanospike array.

3.4 Conclusions

A biomimetics image retrieval platform that is based on a visualization-based image retrieval scheme, has been presented. For overcoming the problem of the limitation of traditional image retrieval engines, which is caused by the difference of terminologies in different study fields, our platform visualizes all of the SEM images in a database according to their visual similarities. Since visual characteristics of nanostructures in SEM images are similar to each other, we can perform inter-field image retrieval even if the similar images belong to different study fields.

As stated before, biomimetics needs close collaboration with different study fields for achieving innovations. Researchers in each study field tend to perform their study within their own community, making inter-field communication difficult. It is also difficult to connect researchers in different study fields. Our retrieval platform provides new opportunities for overcoming these obstacles.

References

1. Shimomura M. (2010). The new trends in next generation biomimetics material technology: learning from biodiversity. *Science & Technology Trends Quarterly Review, 37*, 53–75.

2. Shimomura M. (2012). Engineering biomimetics: integration of biology and nanotechnology, in Design for Innovative Value towards a Sustainable Society: Proceedings of EcoDesign 2011: 7th International Symposium on Environmentally Conscious Design and Inverse Manufacturing, pp. 905–907.

3. Haseyama M., Ogawa T., Takahashi S., Nomura S., Shimomura M. (2017). Biomimetics image retrieval platform, *IEICE Transactions on Information and Systems*, **E100-D**(8), 1563–1573.

4. Kozaki K., Mizoguchi R. (2014). A keyword exploration for retrieval from biomimetics databases. *Joint International Semantic Technology Conference*, 361–377.

5. Schmidhuber J. (2015). Deep learning in neural networks: an overview. *Neural Networks*, **61**, 85–117.

6. Russakovsky O., Deng J., Su H., Krause J., Satheesh S., Ma S., Huang Z., Karpathy A., Khosla A., Bernstein M., Berg A. C., Fei-Fei L. (2015). Imagenet large scale visual recognition challenge. *International Journal of Computer Vision*, **115**(3), 211–252.

7. Gantz J., Chute C., Manfrediz A., Minton S., Reinsel D., Schlichting W., et al. (2008). *The Diverse and Exploding Digital Universe*, IDC White Paper, IDC.

8. Gantz J., Reinsel D. (2010). The Digital Universe Decade, Are You Ready?, IDC iView.

9. IDC Digital Universe Study, sponsored by EMC, December 2012, http://www.emc.com/about/news/press/2012/20121211-01.htm.

10. Haseyama M., Ogawa T., Yagi N. (2013). A review of video retrieval based on image and video semantic understanding. *ITE Transactions on Media Technology and Applications*, **1**(1), 2–9.

11. Haseyama M., Murata T., Ukawa H. (2009). *A New Image Retrieval Interface and its Practical use in "View Search Hokkaido"*, The 13th IEEE International Symposium on Consumer Electronics, pp. 851–852.

12. Haseyama M., Ogawa T. (2013). Trial realization of human-centered multimedia navigation for video retrieval. *International Journal of Human-Computer Interaction*, **29**(2), 96–109.

13. Haseyama M. (2016). Realization of Associative Image Search: development of Image Retrieval Platform for Enhancing Serendipity, 2016 IEEE 46th International Symposium on Multiple-Valued Logic (ISMVL), pp. 56–59.

14. Watanabe T., Haseyama M. (2007). A study on accurate image clustering using color edges. *IEICE Technical Report*, **106**(534), 7–10 (in Japanese).

15. Tokumoto R., Haseyama M. (2007). *Color Distribution-based Similar Image Clustering and its Performance Evaluation*. International Conference on Kansei Engineering and Emotion Research 2007 (KEER2007), vol. C-25.

16. Hirai Y., Yabu H., Matsuo Y., Ijiro K., Shimomura M. (2010). Biomimetic bi-functional silicon nanospike-array structures prepared by using self-organized honeycomb templates and reactive ion etching. *Journal of Materials Chemistry*, **20**(48), 10804–10808.

Chapter 4

Theory of Inventive Problem-Solving Method (TRIZ) Applying Biomimetics

Takeshi Yamauchi,[a] Hidetoshi Kobayashi,[b] and Toru Kobayashi[c]

[a]*Department of Materials Science and Technology,*
Niigata University, 8050, Ikarashi 2-nocho, Nishi-ku,
Niigata 950-2181, Japan
[b]*Department of Mechanical Science and Bioengineering,*
Osaka University, 1-1 Machikaneyama,
Toyonaka 560-0043, Osaka, Japan
[c]*Graduate School of Engineering,*
Division of Electrical Engineering and Computer Science,
Nagasaki University, 1-14 Bunkyo, Nagasaki 852-8521,
Nagasaki, Japan

yamauchi@gs.niigata-u.ac.jp

4.1 Introduction

In recent years, researchers have been stepping up their work on biomimetics, a field focused on introducing high-efficiency and-performance biofunctions into material design [1]. More and more articles on biomimetic engineering have been reported every year, and expectations that the industry will develop practical applications for such are likewise on the rise. Numerous

---

Biomimetics: Connecting Ecology and Engineering by Informatics
Edited by Akihiro Miyauchi and Masatsugu Shimomura
Copyright © 2023 Jenny Stanford Publishing Pte. Ltd.
ISBN 978-981-4968-10-2 (Hardcover), 978-1-003-27717-0 (eBook)
www.jennystanford.com

well-known applications of biomimetics may be cited such as self-cleaning paints based on lotus leaves, easy-to-peel-off tapes inspired by the microstructures in the soles of a gecko's foot, nonreflective films structured like the compound eyes of a moth, shark skin-patterned high-speed swimwear, and labels that use the structural colors of the morpho butterfly. The ranks of companies whose interest in developing materials based on biomimetic engineering principles sparked by news reports about such developments likewise has been increasing. That said, there are more than 7.8 million species of living beings in the world, with an enormous number of different functions and behaviors. Whatever biofunction attracts our attention, it is unclear as to which ones will be useful toward developing new technologies and materials and lead to an optimal material design. In short, most engineers and researchers find themselves vexed by their inability to home in on a single target owing to the excess of options. Thus, case-by-case material design is the mainstream by biomimetic engineering in present-day. Only a portion of the limitless number of biofunctions are being put to use, and there are no effective means for digging out those technological elements that may be necessary. Furthermore, with the International Standardization Organization (ISO) currently studying a variety of regulations with regard to biomimetic engineering, there is demand for biomimetic products to be created that conform to international standards. According to ISO specifications, developing biomimetic biometric products requires they go through the following process: (1) identify issues with existing technologies and materials, (2) search for biofunctions that can resolve those issues, (3) extract and generalize the principles behind the biofunctions that have been discovered, and (4) create and optimize new technologies and materials. The question also arises of the best approach to take for identifying functions among the 7.8 million living things said to exist and for optimizing them. In this chapter, we introduce Theory of Inventive Problem Solving (TRIZ) applying biomimetics and our database called "Biomimetics-Integrating problem- and function-oriented approaches applying TRIZ" which support to create biomimetics products according to ISO specifications.

4.2 Current Conditions Regarding Patents for Biomimetics

The Japan Patent Office's *Survey Report on Technology Trends in Patent Applications* gives us a picture of current tendencies in regard to patents focused on biofunctions [2]. It can be inferred from a review of the data for those products that are mainly related to biomimetics that at present the number of instances in which a patent has been commoditized is limited regardless of country or region. The main products can be broken down as belonging to one the following three broad categories:

(1) Products related to molecules and materials. Examples include hydrophilic and hydrophobic materials (e.g., water-repellent paints, tile-related building materials, and water-repellent glass); structural coloration materials (e.g., chemical fibers); optical materials (e.g., antireflective film and displays); adhesive and gummed materials (e.g., adhesive tape, carpet tile, and cyclone vacuum cleaners); medical and biocompatible materials (e.g., injection needles and cosmetics); low-value resistance and low-friction materials (e.g., competition swimwear, fuselage paint for airplanes, and ship-coating materials); and antifouling materials (e.g., antifouling coating for ship bottoms).

(2) Products meant to reduce the resistivity of a structure (e.g., cooling fans, washing machines, mixers, and the shape of the noses on bullet trains) or save weight (e.g., automobile wheels).

(3) Products related to robots (e.g., robots patterned after dragonflies, elephant noses, etc.) or machine controls (e.g., sensors and software for controlling smart grids).

In Japan, we find numerous products related to the molecular and materials fields such as hydrophilic and hydrophobic materials, optical materials, and adhesive and gummed materials. In the west, in contrast, we encounter products in the machine field. Much work was once being done in Japan in the areas of biomimetic chemistry and robotics, and the country was a leader in molecular scale biomimetics. However, researchers and engineers have not been able to get a grasp on the new currents that emerged in material-related biomimetics in this century. Broadly speaking, this is because in Japan collaborations between different fields as biology and engineering never take place owing to preconceptions in Japanese research and academic settings about interdisciplinary interactions.

Additionally, it is believed that the materials field will become the primary destination for applications of biomimetics. If more products are to be brought to market in these areas, it will be necessary to develop even more technologies in the area of microstructure fabrication techniques in order to reduce manufacturing costs and improve durability. Furthermore, if the biomimetics market is to expand, would-be producers will need to adopt a "biomimetic" way of thinking in the control and processing fields. In particular, observers have highlighted the importance of autonomous distributed control systems, and the expectations of people involved in the field for advances in the development and practical application of such systems are high.

4.3 Engineering Problem Solving Method (TRIZ) Applying Biomimetics

4.3.1 TRIZ Method

There are a variety of approaches that one can take to solving engineering problems. Researchers and engineers have found success in wielding such approaches as a strength, weaknesses, opportunities, and threats (SWOT) analysis, which applies a business framework to the problem; "logic" (or "issue") trees; Osborn's checklist; mind maps; quality control methodology; and the Taguchi method. Among these methods is one that has been applied in a variety of fields since 1990 as a means for generating ideas for material design in mechanical engineering. This is the Theory of Inventive Problem Solving, usually known by its Russian acronym TRIZ (Teoriya Resheniya Izobreatatelskikh Zadach). TRIZ was developed by Genrikh Saulovich Altshuller (1926–1998), who worked as a clerk in a Russian patent office [3–7]. Altshuller came up with TRIZ as a set of "principles for performing creative problem solving" that put a system to the regularities he uncovered in his examinations of some 1.5 million patents. The distinguishing feature of this method is that it presents a set of rules and principles for solving issues in engineering technology. 40 principles for problem-solving is one of problem-solving techniques in TRIZ, a technique to settle a problem from an invention principle of 40 by an inconsistent matrix way. The merit of the TRIZ method is that it presents a set of rules and principles for solving issues in engineering technology. This it does by looking for the patterns in the problems for which solutions are being sought, thus making it possible to get ideas about how to solve those problems regardless of one's field of research. There is any number of ways to apply it based for example on principles, predictions, or effects. Here, we will focus on problem-solving methods that make effective use of the 40 problem-solving principles the theory proposes. The principle-based approach entails taking the physical characteristics spanning the 39 parameters shown on Table 4.1 and using them to create a 39-by-39 matrix comprising "parameters wish to improve" and "problems that will arise when improvement is made (Tables 4.1 and 4.2). The goal is to resolve the technological contradictions represented by the intersections between those parameters an inventor seeks to improve and those parameters that will change for the worse.

Table 4.1 Thirty-nine features of Altshuller's contradiction matrix

1	Weight of mobile object	16	Time of action of a stationary object	31	Harmful factors developed by an object
2	Weight of stationary object	17	Temperature	32	Manufacturability
3	Length of mobile object	18	Brightness	33	Convenience of use
4	Length of stationary object	19	Energy spent by a moving object	34	Repairbility
5	Area of mobile object	20	Energy spent by a stationary object	35	Adaptability
6	Area of stationary object	21	Power	36	Complexity of device
7	Volume of mobile object	22	Loss of energy	37	Complexity of control
8	Volume of stationary object	23	Loss of a substrate	38	Level of automation

(*Continued*)

Table 4.1 (*Continued*)

9	Speed	24	Loss of an information	39	Capacity/productivity
10	Force	25	Loss of time		
11	Tension/pressure	26	Amount of substrate		
12	Shape	27	Reliability		
13	Stability of composition	28	Accuracy of measurement		
14	Strength	29	Accuracy of manufacturing		
15	Time of action of a moving object	30	Harmful factors acting on an object from outside		

Table 4.2 The 40 problem-solving principles of TRIZ

1	Segmentation	16	Partial or excessive action	31	Porous material
2	Extraction	17	Transition into a new dimension	32	Changing the color
3	Local quality	18	Mechanical vibration	33	Homogeneity
4	Asymmetry	19	periodic action	34	Reject and regenerating parts
5	Consolidation	20	Continuity of useful action	35	Transformation of properties
6	Universality	21	Rushing through	36	Phase transition
7	Nesting	22	Convert harm into benefit	37	Thermal expansion
8	Counterweight	23	Feedback	38	Accelerated oxidation
9	Prior counteraction	24	Mediator	39	Inert environment
10	Prior action	25	Self service	40	Composite materials
11	Cushion in advance	26	Copying		
12	Equipotentiality	27	Dispose		
13	Do it in reverse	28	Replacement of mechanical system		
14	Spheroidality	29	Pneumatic hydraulic construction		
15	Dynamicity	30	Flexible membrane or thin film		

4.3.2 Bio-TRIZ Method

Bio-TRIZ is a new concept put forth by former University of Bath professor Julian F. V. Vincent and his associates, and it can solve technical problem to bring high-efficiency biofunctions found in nature into TRIZ's 40 problem-solving principles [8–11]. For example, in metallurgical and mechanical engineering, to open pores in a material means reducing its strength. However, living things create sophisticated structures that prevent cracks from forming when they open pores. This maintains the strength of a material while simultaneously saving weight. Biofunctions in this way are a gold mine for patentable new technologies. They imply ideas for the development of next-generation materials and can also be expected to do much in the area of education in new engineering design. Developing next-generation materials demands their creators to consider the factors as harmonizing with nature, environmental friendliness, and the use of biomass among others. Moreover, they get adapting functions as the diversity to survive against environmental change on the earth. Engineers would like to add the functions in case of materials design for superior performance, however creatures keep the principle to sacrifice something to get new functions as evolution. This optimization concept is called a trade-off. The trade-off is situational decision that involves diminishing or losing one quality, quantity or property of a set or design in return for gains in other aspects. Vilfredo Pareto (1848–1923), Italian engineer and economist, who focused the concept of trade-off in his studies of economic efficiency and income distribution. He discovered Pareto efficiency which is a situation that cannot be modified to make any one individual or preference criterion better off without making at least one individual or preference criterion worse off. He also defined Pareto frontier which is the set of parameterizations that are all Pareto efficient. Finding Pareto frontiers is particularly useful in engineering. By yielding all of the potentially optimal solutions, a designer can make focused the trade-offs of factor 1 (F_1) and factor 2 (F_2) within this constrained set of parameters, rather than needing to consider the full ranges of parameters [12]. The TRIZ method is a kind of problem-solving method using the trade-off and the bio-TRIZ achieves to produce engineering solution adapting global environment on Pareto frontier (Fig. 4.1) [13].

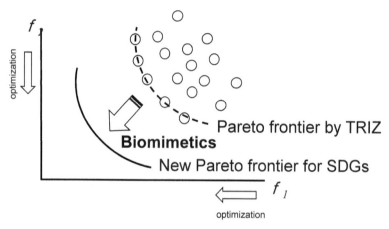

Figure 4.1 Role of biomimetics for optimization between factor 1 and factor 2 in bio-TRIZ.

4.3.3 Examples of Solutions to Technological Contradictions

Next, let us consider an example of how to use the bio-TRIZ which can assist even non-specialist researchers when invent materials in next-generation. There are a lot of patents on materials taking structures of living things on board. One technological contradiction commonly occurs in material-developments in a variety of fields is a requirement to reduce a weight of a material while not reducing such as energy efficiency, power and/or operating time. One example of how to solve this kind of contradiction using a TRIZ principle can be found in our own research which improving the functionality of polymeric actuators.

People working in a variety of fields highly hope for employing conductive polymers as soft actuators that can be operated in low voltages. However, the required amounts of materials and the energy to drive the actuators grows dramatically with the scale-up. While at the same time, reducing a weight causes a problem in mechanical strength. Putting this technological contradiction into the TRIZ contradiction matrix reveals four inventive principles that are effective for solving it as follows: (12) Equipotentiality, (18) Mechanical vibration, (31) Porous materials, and (36) Phase transitions. For example, we can find Patent and Utility Model Number 2010-252422 for a voltage actuator disclosed by Seiko Epson Corporation that enable high-efficiency driving in the filed patents that resolved this technological problem from an engineering point of view. Principle 18 on mechanical vibration was used to develop an actuator equipped with piezoelectric elements that have the resonance frequencies of the lateral and anti-resonance vibrations as the frequency for the drive signal.

Shifting our view to living things, we find that the porous structure in spines of hedgehog or porcupine makes them extremely lightweight and firm. In short, they make skillful use of porous structures. This led the development of an actuator to use a porous structure. While there are many patents associated with porous structures similar to those of living things, there are few proposed solutions related to manufacturing processes for opening the pores in materials because of losing the strength of the materials. The limited examples on materials with artificially opening the holes would include the structures with foam or cell. Foams based on polymeric materials have widespread applications: protective materials such as foamed polyurethane and styrene foam, as well as batteries, fuel cells, filters, lightweight structural materials, thermal insulation, and vibration-proofing materials. However, the pores are often produced irregularly in the manufacturing process and difficult to control the pore size and distribution. One example of manufacturing process for regular porous polymers has been developed using a silica crystal as a mold. In this process, the silica is removed after the polymer is formed. This method requires large amounts of thermal energy to create the silica. Furthermore, chemicals are used to remove the silica from the composite, and high temperatures are required to achieve a phase transition in silica. However, plants of the gramineae produce silica internally at normal temperatures. They absorb silicates from the soil, which then crystallize. The reasons for this are believed to be the strength of the fibers and the lighting effects, i.e., the ease with which light is absorbed by this glass.

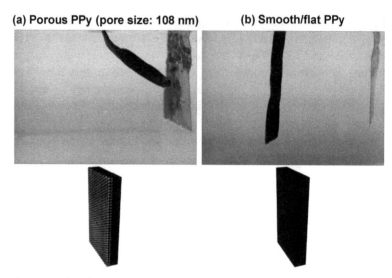

Figure 4.2 Bending motion of soft actuators of poly pyrrole (PPy) film (applied electric potential: 3V). (a) Porous material structure (b) Smooth/flat structure.

Underwater florae also make use of this sort of effective phase transition. For example, agar—a component of seaweed—uses potassium in seawater to easily shift back and forth between sol and gel states, and thus helps to fix a position of the seaweed in the water not to be flown away. We studied making a porous conductive polymer by taking advantage of the phase transition phenomenon in agar to create gel beads. In our synthesizing process, the beads were arranged as molds in the conductive polymer. The beads melted at a temperature of 80°C after compounding. We developed new actuator taking into account the principle of phase transition create a polypyrrole/agar microparticle membrane based on the electrochemical method of polymerization. The obtained membrane is then dipped in an ion exchanged water at 90°C and the microparticles of agar are removed. As a result, the porous polypyrrole membrane was obtained. This porous conductive polymer membrane is approximately 9 μm thick and has the average pore diameter of 108 nm. The actuation behavior of the porous membrane and the smooth/flat membrane are shown in Fig. 4.2. The porous membrane displays a relatively large bending motion compared to the smooth/flat one. Furthermore, we made porous membranes with a large average pore size (diameter: 293 nm) and evaluated bending motions in the three types of conductive thin films (a smooth/flat membrane, porous membranes with average pore diameters of 108 nm and 293 nm). The bending speeds of each samples were 2.4 deg/s, 20.4 deg/s, and 9.6 deg/s, respectively (see Fig. 4.3). These results suggest that it is possible to control deformation movement and driving speed by the porous structures.

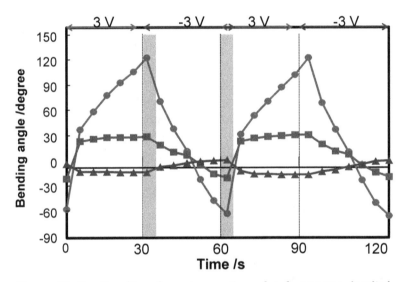

Figure 4.3 Functionality of curving motion of soft actuator (applied electric potential: 3V). (○) Porous material structure (avg. pore dia. 108 nm), (□) Porous material structure (avg. pore dia. 293 nm), (△) Smooth and flat structure.

4.4 Database of Inventive Problem-Solving Method (TRIZ) Applying Biomimetics

4.4.1 Problem-Oriented Approach-Search from Technical Contradiction Matrix

No works in process engineering have been done to find applications using a sophisticated evident in living things. The reason seems to be that even if engineers attempt to find uses in the data of living things, it is extremely difficult to come across data that provides a stimulus for inventions.

It is difficult for engineers, who do not have knowledge of a nature, to get solution for their engineering problems from biomimetics at present time. If they can get a hint for a technological problem automatically, it will be very convenient to produce new products, especially supporting Sustainable Development Goals (SDGs) because the hit is based on nature. We developed database for engineers to find data on living things that will point them in serendipitous directions and facilitate coming up with patents relevant to material design, development processes and systems, and a wide range of other problems.

The strength of this database lies in the fact that when the user queries it over technological contradictions—the problem of improving one parameter having a negative impact on another—it has the framework in place to automatically display any number of biofunctions that might suggest a solution as it runs through the four processes. Our database comprises carefully selected information—stored in files categorized into the 40 TRIZ problem-solving principles—about living things that could be used for coming up with patents.

This database is designed to support users developing ISO-certified biomimetic products to get ideas from nature. There are demands for created biomimetic products to conform the international standards that the ISO currently investigating a variety of regulations on biomimetic engineering. There are 4-steps for developing biomimetic products according to ISO specifications: (1) identify issues with existing technologies and materials, (2) search for biofunctions that can resolve those issues, (3) extract and generalize the principles behind the biofunctions that have been discovered, and (4) create and optimize new technologies and materials. This database can provide novel idea to develop ISO-certified biomimetic products (Fig. 4.4).

The strength of this database lies in the fact that when a user queries the database over technological contradictions, namely a problem of improving one parameter having a negative impact on another. It has the framework in place to automatically display any number of biofunctions that might suggest a solution with the four processes as shown in Fig. 4.5 and 4.6. Our database comprises carefully selected information stored in files categorized into the 40 TRIZ problem-solving principles about living things that could be used for coming up with patents. This database could contribute to a decision making in the creation of biomimetic products. Our database can supply the problem-solving principles that would be appropriate for resolving the issues by merely condensing the technological problems which engineers face and putting them into a contradictions matrix. Furthermore, the database can search out the biofunctions for users. The user can get ideas efficiently for developing biomimetic products in a short period of time by optimizing the biofunctions from this database. Furthermore, the data contained can also contribute to product development based on existing work since the user can also view an inventory of biomimetic products.

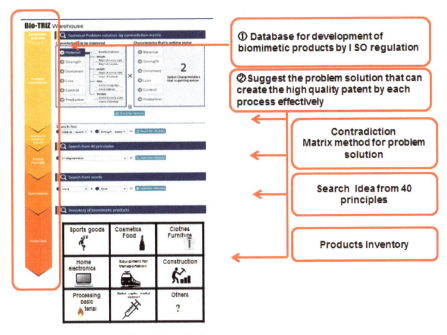

Figure 4.4 An outline of this database.

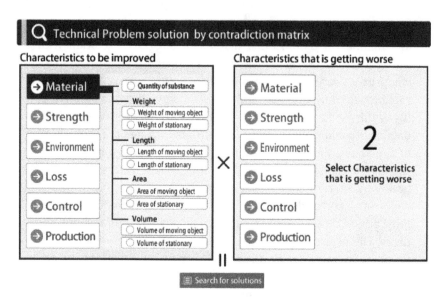

Figure 4.5 Using the contradictions matrix in this database.

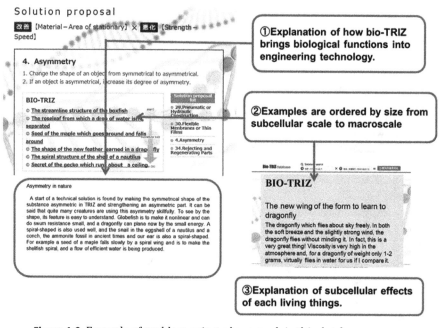

Figure 4.6 Example of problem-oriented approach in this database.

4.4.2 Function-Oriented Approach-Search from Function

Data obtained from a problem-oriented approach is transformed by Resource Description Framework (RDF) which utilizes biomimetic information from a function parameter. This method can search for a natural principle extracted natural phenomenon and a biomimetic solution-guide from 40 principles in TRIZ. Users can get ideas for problem solving with function parameter thorough natural phenomenon and information on bio-TRIZ by a different viewpoint (Fig. 4.7). So, we construct a two-way research process, firstly a "problem-oriented approach" from 39-by-39 matrix and secondly a "function-oriented approach" which can get biomimetic information from the function [14–16]. You choose function which you would like to make act on, and state of the solid, liquid and gas. As shown in Fig. 4.8, you can search for mechanism of a similar creature as well as the natural principle to improve the function.

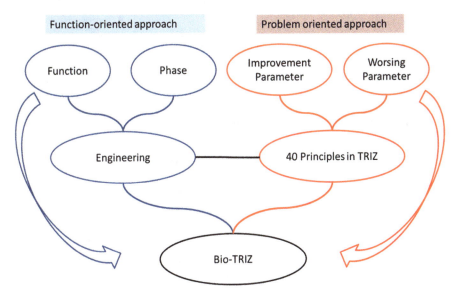

Figure 4.7 Two kinds of search system in the database.

Theory of Inventive Problem-Solving Method Applying Biomimetics

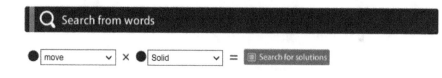

Engineering	Biomimetics	TRIZ principal
friction	The dog which is easy even if I run through a slippery snowy road	4. Asymmetry
brush	If wild burdocks touch, they don't get away!	3. Local Conditions
hyperboloid	Seed of the maple which goes around and falls around	4. Asymmetry
desorption	The ceiling, secret of the gecko which runs about	3. Local Conditions
vibration	A human heart is the pump which are multiple functions.	1. Segmentation
resonance	Secret of 6 legs walking of a cockroach	19. Periodic Action
inertia	The wild goose how isn't which crashed even if it gathers	15. Dynamics
light electrophoresis	Vegetable MARANTA which moves by light	11. Cushion in advance
spiral	The bacterial flagellum motor equipped with a clutch	14. Spheroidality
condensation	Nectar of the aphis which falls by wax	30. Phase Transition
explosion	Jet of octopus	29. Pneumatic or hydraulic Construction
beak effect	Even if it's stuck into a mosquito, it isn't painful.	3. Local Conditions
fluidization	The new wing of the form to learn to dragonfly	15. Dynamics
shape memory effect	Both tree bugs and insect bites "Miura fold"	7. Nesting

Figure 4.8 Example of function-oriented approach in this database.

4.4.3 Inventory of Biomimetic Products

The 2030 Agenda for Sustainable Development, adopted by all United Nations Member States in 2015, provides a shared blueprint for peace and prosperity for people and the planet, now and into the future. At its heart are the 17 SDGs, which are an urgent call for action by all countries—developed and developing—in a global partnership. A successful sustainable development agenda requires partnerships between governments, the private sector and civil society. For more information on what the UN System is doing to achieve Goal 17. Biomimetics is concept that using ideas from nature to further technology, and it can contribute to realize the SDGs goals because nature gives us solution for engineering problem to realize SDGs. This database includes amount of biomimetics products information in various kind industry for SDGs such as materials science, electronics, cosmetics, transformation, sports, constriction, etc.

Our database comprises carefully selected information—stored in files categorized into the 40 TRIZ problem-solving principles—about living things that could be used for coming up with patents. According to ISO specifications, a user can get ideas for efficiently developing biomimetic products in a short period of time by problem-oriented approach and function-oriented approach. Furthermore, the contained data can also contribute to product development based on existing work since the user can also view an inventory of biomimetic products related with SDGs.

4.5 A Motivating Example of Database

4.5.1 Problem-Oriented Approach for Windmills

Let us demonstrate to develop a new windmill for a motivating example. Increasing the surface area of the blades used on the tiny windmills creates a large rotational torque, which allows for obtaining greater energy. However, increasing the surface area makes the rotation slower. This is a contradiction. We use this database to search for inventive principles that would resolve the conflict of surface area versus speed, and the four principles are found. These four principles are based on the TRIZ. Explanations are as follows:

29. Pneumatics or hydraulics

    (1) Using expansion, fluid-filling, air cushions, and other liquid/gas phenomena not found in solids

30. Flexible membranes or thin film

    (1) Using flexible shell and membrane coatings in lieu of three-dimensional shapes

    (2) Isolating objects from the outside environment through use of shells and membranes

4. Asymmetry

    (1) Turning the symmetry of a substance asymmetrical

(2) Strengthening asymmetrical components

34. Rejection and re generation, Discarding and recovering

(1) Exclude elements of an object that have completed their function

(2) Revitalize the consumable elements of an object

When we search for further data in this database, we can get information concerning a new wing form devised from that of dragonflies, corresponding to the principle 4.

Asymmetry. Specifically, a cross section of the wings of dragonflies reveals that, unlike those of hawks and kites, they are not a streamlined form; instead, they have a corrugated structure, creating small eddies of air at their tips and conveying air on the exterior smoothly toward the back of the wings, allowing the dragonfly to achieve lift even amidst minor gusts of wind. The proposed solution of using a wing design inspired by dragonflies makes use of the above structure. This database is being used to provide a high quality of potential solutions. The database also contains different biological data within the principle 4. Asymmetry (see below), so the researcher can make a reference to these varying data points and use their technological prowess to develop and patent new biomimetic technologies. A few examples are as follows:

"Hovering movements of hummingbird wings"

Birds obtain lift by pushing their wings downward and use this to fly. Insects gain lift commensurate to the degree to which they flap their wings. Hummingbirds are somewhere between insects and birds. They obtain 75% of their buoyancy by beating their wings down and 25% when they draw them up.

"Twirling maple seeds"

When maple seeds rotate, small eddies at their tips allow air pressure near the top of the blades to decrease and pump the blades up, causing them to remain in flight.

4.5.2 Function-Oriented Approach for Windmills

In a function-oriented approach, we identify that most existing wind turbines have streamlined blades that resemble those of hawks and kites, with the physical size of the blade increasing. We thus search for a combination of "move X solid." As seen below, there were 14 hits for natural principles that can be used to resolve this issue (see Fig. 4.8). Friction, brush, hyperbolic-conchoid, attaching-detaching, vibration, resonance, inertia, photopheresis, spiral, condensation, explosion, beak effect, fluidization, shape memory effect. If we consider that controlling the flow of wind is important, here, "fluidization" is a crucial element. If we filter a word "fluidization", "wings inspired by dragonflies," of the principle 4. Asymmetry is hit. It is interesting that both approaches lead us to the biomimetic data of dragonflies. If we turn to another natural principle of "inertia", "new morphing wings" is hit. We could get an idea of developing morphing wings, which have the following elements: the way in which birds spread their wings widely when they are landing and taking off, and quickly descending on their prey. They can also fold their wings tight to reduce a wind resistance. In this way, both approaches allow for arriving at a substantive method of problem-solving, and one can obtain different knowledge from the biological world for the production of new patents. The reader will see how this technique supports a unique thought process.

4.5.3 Inventory of Biomimetic Products for Windmills

Examples of domestic and foreign patents on various fields of industry such as materials science, electronics, cosmetics, transformation, sports, can be figured out from this database. We can search patents of biomimetic products by the optimization of our new idea. You can get information about windmills in electronics. An aerial gap is set up to the aspect of the wing, aerial resistance is suppressed and a smooth aerial flow is invented like a wing of a dragonfly. SHARP Co. adopted the dragonfly-like wing to their air-conditioner and slim ion fan and a slim ion fan. The wind generated by these fan flows smoothly and the resistance was suppressed. The problem-oriented and function-oriented approach of new windmill-fan is summarized in Table 4.3.

Table 4.3 Information for development of new windmills from this database

ISO specifications	Problem-oriented approach	Function-oriented approach
(1) Identify issues with existing technologies and materials	Surface area vs speed	Move X Solod
(2) Search for biofunctions that can resolve those issues	Dragonfly	Dragonfly
(3) Extract and generalize the principles behind the biofunctions that have been discovered	Asymmetry	Fuidization
(4) Create and optimize new technologies and materials		

Product	Air cleaner
Brand name	S-style
Manufacturing firm	Sharp
Corporation	(Osaka, Japan)

4.6 Conclusion

As noted in the foregoing, we have introduced the engineering problem-solving method applying biomimetics, and explored the possibilities of bringing the wonders of living things into engineering. Biofunctions comprise a gold mine of technologies to be patented. The researcher or inventor who can out those biofunctions, work out the regularities submerged within, and skillfully wield those findings like a winning chess piece should be able to help come up with new designs in engineering. It is our belief that by making the most of the database for the engineering problem-solving method applying biomimetics, individuals involved in research at companies whatever the field will be able to come up with fresh ideas for resolving technological contradictions unlike those that have already led to patenting efforts. It will also help them to take advantage of the engineering technologies at companies that in the past backed up the work of industries, and as a result of these various applications they will produce new technologies that will create the new industries for future.

References

1. Among numerous works, we can single out Shimomura M, Seibutsu no tayôsei ni manabu shinsedai: baiomimetikku zairyô gijutsu no shinchôryô [A new generation learns from the diversity of life: New currents in biomimetic materials technology], *Science & Technology Trends*, 2010, 9–27.

2. Japan Patent Office [JPO]. *Tokkyo Shutsugan Gijutsu Dôkô Chôsa Hôkokusho* [Survey report on technology trends in patent applications], JPO, 2015, 39.

3. Altshuller G. S. *Creativity as an Exact Science: The Theory of the Solution of Inventive Problems* (trans. by Anthony Williams), Gordon and Breach Science Publishers, 1984, 1–223.

4. Sawaguchi M. *VE to TRIZ* [VE and TRIZ], Dôyűkan, 2002, 56–153.

5. Kasai H. *Kaihatsu Sekkei no Tame no TRIZ Nyűmon* [An Introduction to TRIZ for Development Design], JUSE Press, 2006, 35–175. Webb B., Consi T. R. Eds. *Biorobotics, Methods & Applications*. AAAI Press/The MIT Press, London, 2001, ISBN: 026273141X, Pages 250.

6. Kasuya S. *Zukai—kore de Tsukaeru: TRIZ/USIT* [Visual guides—With this you can use it: TRIZ-USIT], Japan Management Association Management Center, 2006, 15–74. Claus M., Kubler H. *Wood—The Internal Optimization of Trees*, Springer Verlag, Heidelberg, 2. Auflage1997.

7. Hasebe M. et al. *Hajimeyô Kantan TRIZ* [Let's begin—TRIZ made simple], Nikkan Kôgyô Shinbun, Ltd., 2007.

8. Vincent J. F. V., Mann D. *Baiomimetikkusu Handobukku* [Handbook of Biomimetics], trans. OSADA Yoshihito, NTS Inc., 2000, 3–14.

9. Vincent J. F. V. *Baiomimetikkusu no Shintenkai* [New Developments in Biomimetics], NTS Inc., 2002, 9–25.

10. Vincent J. F. V., Mann D. TRIZ in biology teaching. *TRIZ Journal*, September 2000.

11. Mann D. Integrating knowledge from biology into the TRIZ framework. *TRIZ Journal*, October 2001.

12. Costa N. R., Lourenco J. A. Exploring pareto frontiers in the response surface methodology, in *Transactions on Engineering Technologies: World Congress on Engineering 2014* (Yang G.-C., Ao S.-I., Gelman L., eds), Springer, Berlin/Heidelberg, 2015, pp. 399–412.

13. Vincent J. F. V. The trade-off: a central concept for biomimetics. *Bioinspired, Biomimetics, Nanobiomimetics,* 2016, 1-10.

14. Kobayashi T., Isono Y., Arai K., Yamauchi T., Kobayashi H. Bio-TRIZ database for sustainable lifestyle-technology transfer from nature to engineering, *Proceedings-International Electronics Symposium on Knowledge Creation and Intelligent Computing,* 2017, pp. 284–288.

15. Kobayashi T., Isono Y., Yamauchi T., Kobayashi H. Serendipity-oriented Bio-TRIZ database for sustainable lifestyle, in *Proceedings of 10th International Symposium on Nature-Inspired Technology,* 2017, p. 17.

16. Isono Y., Yamauchi T., Kobayashi H., Kobayashi T. *Proceedings of 5th Nagoya Biomimetics International Symposium,* 2016, p. 46.

Chapter 5

Urban Planning by Learning from Living Creatures

Mamoru Taniguchi

Faculty of Engineering, Information and Systems,
Department of Policy and Planning Sciences,
University of Tsukuba, 1-1-1 Tennodai, Tsukuba-City 305-8573, Japan

mamoru@sk.tsukuba.ac.jp

5.1 Introduction

Living creatures and cities are similar: roads resemble blood vessels; houses and offices have much in common with cells; arterial roads can be compared to the aorta; fine alleys can be compared to capillaries. In addition, both living creatures and cities must consume energy to continue their activities. They all generate waste. Furthermore, they "grow up," "metabolize," "attempt to be healthy," "become sick," "sustain injury," "heal," "age," "regenerate," and "evolve." When comparing the two in this way, in fact, many aspects are similar. Learning from living things can provide remedies for troubled cities.

Although it has long been pointed out that such cities and creatures are similar, such examinations are all aimed at growing cities. In contrast, this report is the first to describe application

---

Biomimetics: Connecting Ecology and Engineering by Informatics
Edited by Akihiro Miyauchi and Masatsugu Shimomura
Copyright © 2023 Jenny Stanford Publishing Pte. Ltd.
ISBN 978-981-4968-10-2 (Hardcover), 978-1-003-27717-0 (eBook)
www.jennystanford.com

of biomimetics to various urban problems that occur during a period of population decline. Particularly in countries, such as Japan, where cities have matured, as discussed in this chapter, inconveniences equivalent to aging and lifestyle-related diseases are prevalent when viewed as living organisms. Every city needs a local physician, such as a family doctor, who can take care of their symptoms. However, specialists who can meet such needs do not yet exist in sufficient quantity or quality. In many cities, various incorrect prescriptions are made based on beliefs of amateurs. For that reason, urban illnesses are not being ameliorated or cured. This chapter presents some referential examples of what wisdom can be obtained from living creatures to cure lifestyle-related diseases in cities.

5.2 Urban Growth and Analogy to Living Creatures

Apparently, *Cities in Evolution*, which Patrick Geddes wrote in 1915, first introduced the perspective of biomimetics in urban planning [1]. Since then, the approaches from the biological perspective in urban planning have not been many. Some prominent urban planning masters such as Lewis Mumford and Ebenezer Howard have applied biological analyses to cities. To date, masters such as Geddes, Mumford, and Howard have put forth a biomimetic perspective in urban development, but all adopt the perspective of a city's biological expansion and evolution in a growing world. Nevertheless, in Japan today, the times have already changed rapidly and starkly. We are entering an era of population decline. Along with this, various lifestyle-related diseases that did not exist in the past have developed on the scale of cities. Details of this idea are summarized below.

5.3 Cities Affected by Lifestyle-Related Diseases

5.3.1 Metabolic Syndrome (Obesity)

This section gives an explanation of "disease" when regarding city as a living creature. Particularly in cities where maturity has progressed after a certain period of growth, we can organize our observations from a broad perspective that phenomena similar to those of lifestyle-related diseases, namely adult diseases, in humans, occur on a larger scale in various cities.

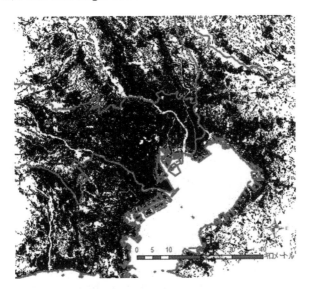

Figure 5.1 Tokyo Metropolitan Area (2014). The black areas represent urbanized built-up areas. National Land Information Division, Ministry of Land, Infrastructure, Transport and Tourism: National Land Numerical Information Download Service http://nlftp.mlit.go.jp/ksj/other/faq.html. Last view 2018/01/10.

First, how large an area must be covered for each city to support urban activities? For example, in huge cities such as Tokyo, suburban residential areas extend far from the city center (Fig. 5.1). As this figure depicts, the urban area is not completely continuous from the city center to the suburbs. The actual situation is that farmland and vacant land are spreading among urbanized areas. The term "sprawl" is used to describe this situation. Unfortunately, Japanese cities have strong private ownership and tend to be lightly planned. For those reasons, efficient urban areas have not formed. Although population declines have already begun in many metropolitan areas, some cases exist in which new homes are still being constructed in suburbs. Looking at how these urban areas expand spatially, the facilities are not slim to fit the space necessary for a city. Therefore, the city structure spreads inefficiently. In summary, large cities in Japan exhibit effects similar to those of metabolic syndrome: they can be characterized as obese.

5.3.2 Hypertension

The influences of obesity appear in circulatory systems. Sprawling urban areas adversely affected by metabolic syndrome are areas that are not fully prepared for urban planning. In such places, urban infrastructure such as roads is often not provided properly. Even if the city is extended widely into the suburbs, traffic congestion will occur in various places unless a road network is prepared as a suitable urban structure. The traffic congestion point is a kind of blood clot. A situation in which high pressure is always applied to the traffic network is similar to hypertension in humans.

Various road maintenance entities, such as the national government and local governments, correspond to blood vessels. Nevertheless, the role of each local government, such as municipalities, is to decide the plan of the local transportation network. Transportation networks such as roads are not closed only by local governments. A transportation network can only function effectively if wide-area seamless connections exist. For this reason, it is probably worth confirming whether a well-connected transportation network is planned between local governments from a regional perspective beyond local governments. Figure 5.2 shows the master plan city structure map of each municipality in Fukuoka prefecture, pasted together to form a single map.

Fukuoka prefecture, an advanced prefecture, is promoting wide-area town planning that is not confined to the boundaries of municipalities. However, this mosaic chart shows the situation in which one is planning only within the scope of one's own municipality, but given positions of the respective municipalities. If each city, town, or village has a different concept of network hierarchy, then it is apparent that many of them are not connected at the border. To prevent blood clots from forming at the boundaries of municipalities, one must take a plan when viewing the entire wide-area urban area, as a body.

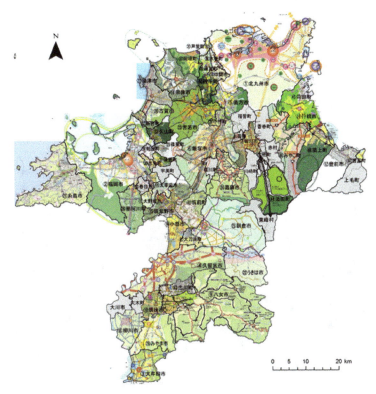

Figure 5.2 Network and core area plan for each municipality in Fukuoka Prefecture [2].

5.3.3 Osteoporosis

In recent years, vacant houses and vacant lots have increased both in the city center and in the suburbs (Fig. 5.3). They progress in various places without being noticed. Nobody noticed that anything has changed with a few more empty houses. However, if the symptoms progress to a certain level, then various services such as shops and public transportation cannot be maintained in the area. Such a case corresponds morphologically to osteoporosis.

5.3.4 Cancer

As the population declines, cities must reduce their size. However, there are some cases where they are expanding uncontrollably.

For example, in suburban new towns that were built during high growth, many old housing complexes are in need of renewal. This is a so-called old new town problem. In response to these issues, low-rise and middle-rise residential areas (Fig. 5.4) are often rebuilt into high-rise residences; in some cases, tower-type condominiums are built (Fig. 5.5).

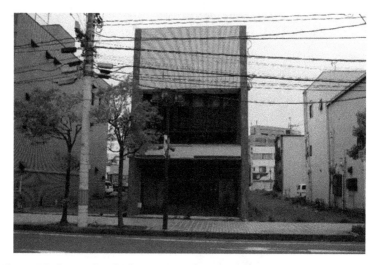

Figure 5.3 A town in which osteoporosis is progressing.

Ways to increase this capacity exist because the cost of this single rebuilding will be covered in this rebuilding project. Therefore, the floor area that can be sold will be increased. The proceeds of the sale will be used to finance the project. This mechanism is not sustainable. When such an expansion-type redevelopment is promoted in an area with population shrinkage, the depressed symptoms of the entire metropolitan area will be worsened. Of course, it is natural for private companies to take action to earn profits. As long as this method is used, the impetus to increase building capacity is powerful: Can this be regarded as oncogenesis? Does it resemble the formation of cancer cells?

An important difficulty is that such a runaway system which promotes cancerous growth is recommended based on the evaluation that the private sector's vitality is improved from a short-sighted perspective. In the future, the population is expected to continue declining, but will the next round of rebuilding be intended to make buildings even higher with larger capacity?

The cases described herein are just a few examples of cities that are exhibiting lifestyle-related decay. In the following, while particularly addressing the pattern of cell death, future urban development is described.

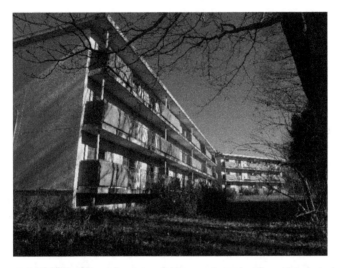

Figure 5.4 Old "New Town" apartment house that must be regenerated.

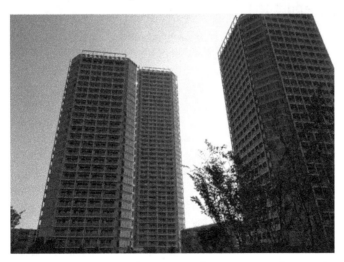

Figure 5.5 Tower-type condominiums that increase the number of households drastically.

5.4 Using Apoptosis (Programmed Cell Death) in Urban Planning

5.4.1 Two Patterns of Cell Death

As urban planning benefits from patterns exhibited by living creatures, it can be useful to understand different patterns of cell death. Two are generally known as "apoptosis" and "necrosis." Apoptosis is a planned cell death that has been programmed in advance to keep the body healthy. In the process, the cell itself shrinks and breaks down. It is then absorbed by surrounding cells. The dead matter is finally processed cleanly. Therefore, cell death does not bother surrounding cells and has no adverse effect on the whole organism. Necrosis is unexpected cell death caused by injury or illness. Specifically, the cells themselves become necrotic. The cell contents leak, causing inflammation and suppuration. It can be said that necrosis afflicts a city that has been devastated by disasters. One might infer that the foundation of city planning is to prepare for such unexpected necrosis under usual conditions.

5.4.2 Compact Town Development Learned from Apoptosis

An easy-to-understand example of apoptosis is the experience of a fetus. In fact, all people had webbed fingers of the hand during their fetal stage of development. However, when born, such webs had already disappeared. The web that appears temporarily and then disappears during fetal growth is a vestige of our ancestors when they were amphibians during the evolutionary process [3]. Cell death that eliminates the web naturally is unmistakably apoptotic. Apoptosis is also a phenomenon by which a tail disappears as a tadpole grows, and in which our skin cells are replaced with new cells within a few months. When such changes occur, the surrounding cells are not adversely affected. This chapter emphasizes this concept of apoptosis because such an idea will function effectively in a society with a declining population. The quiet withdrawal of cells caused by apoptosis is extremely suggestive of creation of a compact city, which is necessary in the era of population decline.

In the metropolitan area of Copenhagen, the capital of Denmark, a plan called a finger plan has been devised and implemented to promote compact urban development. Figure 5.6 shows the basic concept, with the palm in the center of Copenhagen, with spreading fingers toward the suburbs. In the suburbs, growth occurs only in the areas corresponding to the five fingers through which the public transportation axis passes. This is an easy-to-understand expression of the idea of allowing the implementation of urban development. In other words, the portion corresponding to webbing is an easy-to-understand message that urbanization is not recommended.

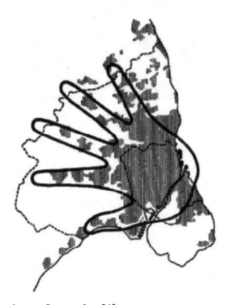

Figure 5.6 Copenhagen finger plan [4].

5.4.3 Necessity of Reduced Diet

The idea of apoptosis is also important for preventing the cancerous growth of cities as described in the previous section. The essence of cancerous growth is that growth should not increase without control. For this reason, the basis for preventing urban cancerous growth is to present as a public policy that what should be reduced is reduced. A typical example of a good practice is the reduction of public housing in Germany.

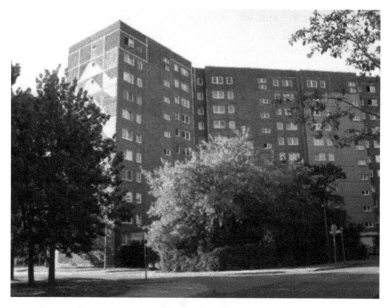

Figure 5.7 Middle-rise housing group (former East Berlin) to be reduced.

In the suburbs of the former East Berlin of Germany, the approximately 10-story medium-rise houses that were supplied in large quantities during the former East Germany period have become obsolete. Many vacant residences have come to exist throughout the area. The security situation has deteriorated. When regenerating the area, instead of rebuilding it into a higher-rise tower-type condominium to promote cancerous growth, the number of houses in each building was reduced drastically. For example, an act called "reduction building" that remodels a middle-rise housing group as shown in Fig. 5.7 into a low-rise apartment building as shown in Fig. 5.8 is being conducted in various places to prevent regional decline. It plays a large role in the process described above. As these photographs clarify, this is an effort to reduce the tasteless and dry mid-rise residential area to small apartments with consideration for the surrounding environment and the design of the building itself. In such cases, it does not consider selling new floors to secure the business: it does not incorporate the mechanism of cancerous growth. Instead, using taxes as a public project, it is possible to implement the project. If it is left unattended as it is, the loss that occurs in the future region is expected to be quite large. It is thought that treating the area as a public project first will lead the area to a more desirable state in the future. The act of systematically reducing the number of cellular activities in a region is similar to apoptosis. Before leaving the area necrotic because of symptoms of necrosis when left unattended, probably the cells were intentionally erased so as not to disturb the surroundings.

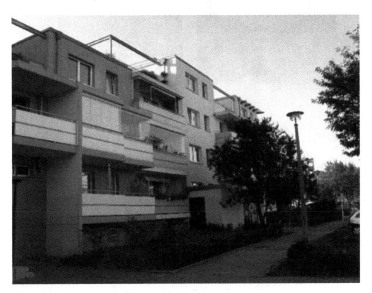

Figure 5.8 Detached housing complex (former East Berlin).

5.4.4 Necessity of District Karte (Patient Chart)

From this series of studies, probably each district should have its own medical chart: a karte (patient chart). The karte must cover basic information such as characteristics of residents and buildings, convenience of public transportation and public facilities in each district (Fig. 5.9). Additionally, it is desirable to augment the karte with information that has been predicted as to what kind of problems might occur in that area over the next 10–20 years. It is important to "visualize" the situation of each district that makes up the city in this way. At the same time, probably it is important to train a city doctor who diagnoses and formulates a prescription for each district based on such records.

102 | Urban Planning by Learning from Living Creatures

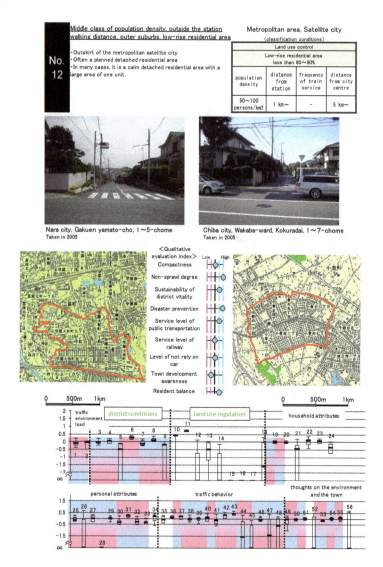

Figure 5.9 Sample of Karte: Patient Chart (district level).

5.5 Concluding Remarks: Thinking about an Evolutionarily Stable Region (ESR)

If a hawk and pigeon are confronted directly, the hawk is clearly stronger. However, whereas pigeons breed steadily everywhere, hawks are often protected and are more likely to become extinct than pigeons. For this reason, pigeons are more evolutionarily stable than hawks. This concept was proposed by Maynard Smith as "evolutionarily stable strategy" [5]. Such relations are applicable to cities and regions as they are. At present, what cities are strong and praised are "economically strong cities (=big cities to earn)?" One can infer that such "economically strong cities" are stronger in a one-on-one game against "loose country towns."

These days, one can expect that such economically strong cities will evolve and strengthen. However, is it really an evolutionary stable strategy for human beings? If one tries to solve the uneconomics of functional agglomeration by further functional agglomeration, it seems to overlap with the figure of a dinosaur that has been destroyed as a result of repeated evolution by enlarging the body. One hopes that cities will not go the way of the *Tyrannosaurus rex* of the past. At the same time, one must ask once again what type of urban system is evolutionarily stable in response to changes in the environment and society. A laid-back country town that seems completely unrelated to the evolution of the city might play a role similar to a small mammal that survived in the shade of a dinosaur. If one borrows a bit of Maynard Smith's words to drop it into a region, one can start exploring "evolutionarily stable regions" [6].

References

1. Geddes P. *Cities in Evolution, An Introduction to the Town Planning Movement and to the Study of Civics*, Williams & Norgate, 1915.

2. Morimoto E., Akahoshi K., Yuki I., Kochi K., Taniguchi M. Fragmented city planning seen from a wide perspective, –a consolidated map of a municipal master plan–. *Journal of Japan Society of Civil Engineers, D3*, **73**(5), 2017, I_345–I_354.

3. Haeckel E., Generelle Morphologie der Organismen, Bd. 2, Verlag von Georg Reimer, 1866.

4. Danish Ministry of Environment. *The Finger Plan: A Strategy for the Development of the Greater Copenhagen Area*, 2015, p. 5.

5. Smith J. M. *Evolution and the Theory of Games*, Cambridge University Press, 1982.

6. Taniguchi M. *Town Development Learned from Living Creatures, -Urban Mitigation Measures in Cities by Biomimetics*, Corona Publishing Co. Ltd., 2018. (in Japanese).

Chapter 6

Functional Elucidation of Biological Interactions in Agricultural Ecosystems and the Application of Biomimetics to Plant Protection

Naoki Mori,[a] Takuma Takanashi,[b] and Hidefumi Mitsuno[c]

[a]*Division of Applied Life Sciences,*
Graduate School of Agricultural Science, Kyoto University, Kyoto, Japan
[b]*Tohoku Research Center,*
Forestry and Forest Products Research Institute, Morioka, Japan
[c]*Research Center for Advanced Science and Technology,*
The University of Tokyo, Tokyo, Japan

mori.naoki.8a@kyoto-u.ac.jp, takanasi@affrc.go.jp, mitsuno@brain.imi.i.u-tokyo.ac.jp

Studies on the biomimetics of the biological interactions in agricultural ecosystems are expected to create more robust, sustainable technologies for plant protection in the long term. We are trying to develop effective strategies to control insect pest behaviors using acoustic and chemical information to enhance plant defense systems of plant trichomes for environmentally friendly plant protection.

Biomimetics: Connecting Ecology and Engineering by Informatics
Edited by Akihiro Miyauchi and Masatsugu Shimomura
Copyright © 2023 Jenny Stanford Publishing Pte. Ltd.
ISBN 978-981-4968-10-2 (Hardcover), 978-1-003-27717-0 (eBook)
www.jennystanford.com

6.1 Vibrational Interactions in Beetles and Bugs and Applications in Plant Protection

6.1.1 Background

Vibrations are essential sources of information that insects utilize during biological interactions. Many insects display a variety of behaviors in response to vibrations. The functional significance of vibration-mediated interactions can be classified into three categories: (i) sexual communication, (ii) social communication, and (iii) predator–prey interactions (e.g., [12, 36]). Although the amount of reports concerning vibrational interactions has increased across a range of insect orders [11, 12, 41], studies of pest species damaging plants remain limited in Hemiptera, Coleoptera, and a few other orders (e.g., Polajnar et al. [23]; Takanashi et al. [36]). In this section, we focus on Coleoptera and Hemiptera (i.e., beetles and bugs, which include several agricultural and forest pests) to review vibrational interactions and their application in plant protection.

6.1.2 Vibrational Interactions in Beetles and Bugs

Vibrational interactions, such as (i) sexual communication, (ii) social communication, and (iii) predator–prey interactions, occur in several families of Coleoptera and Hemiptera [36] (Table 6.1). In Coleoptera, species within the families Anobiidae, Tenebrionidae, and Curculionidae use vibrations to display (i) sexual communication. For example, the deathwatch beetle, *Xestobium rufovillosum* (Anobiidae), taps its head on the substrate, and this behavior enables males to locate females by generating long-range vibrational replies [10]. Across 30 hemipteran families, including the suborders Heteroptera and Auchenorrhyncha, vibrations are used for male courtship and communication between the sexes [36]. *Nezara viridula* adults (Pentatomidae: Heteroptera) produce species- and sex-specific vibrational signals for sexual communication. The signals are often exchanged between the sexes in a duet [3, 4, 22]. Males of the brown planthopper, *Nilaparvata lugens* (Delphacidae: Auchenorrhyncha), track down females that produce vibrations by drumming their abdomens on rice plants [13].

Table 6.1 Vibrational interactions in families of coleopteran beetles and hemipteran bugs as an information source, reported in Takanashi et al. (2019)

	No. of families	
Vibrational interaction	**Coleoptera**	**Hemiptera**
Sexual communication	4	30
Social communication	2	3
Predator–prey interactions	5	4

Vibrations mediate social interactions among adults, larvae, embryos, and pupae in two coleopteran families (Scarabaeidae and Chrysomelidae) and three hemipteran families (Cydnidae, Parastrachiidae, and Pentatomidae) [36] (Table 6.1). In the group-living beetle, *Trypoxylus dichotomus* (Scarabaeidae), larvae freeze in response to vibrations produced by pupal drumming, thereby avoiding and protecting the pupae in the soil [21]. Larval freezing responses to pupae are considered to have evolved from the response to predators because larvae also display freezing responses to vibrations produced by moles digging in the soil [19, 20]. In the brown marmorated stink bug, *Halyomorpha halys* (Pentatomidae), synchronous hatching is induced by a single eggshell-cracking vibration over a short period in a clutch of eggs that are in contact with each other [5, 6]. By contrast, mothers of the subsocial burrower bug, *Adomerus rotundus* (Cydnidae), and the subsocial shield bug, *Parastrachia japonensis* (Parastrachiidae), produce vibrations by shaking their bodies while maintaining an egg-guarding posture [29, 30]. The vibrations promote synchronous hatching, thereby decreasing the probability of sibling cannibalism [31].

Predator–prey interactions occur in five coleopteran families (Tenebrionidae, Chrysomelidae, Cerambycidae, Nitidulidae, and Scarabaeidae) and four hemipteran families (Cydnidae, Reduviidae, Membracidae, and Aphididae) [36]. *Onymacris plana plana* (Tenebrionidae) displays behavioral responses to vibrations, presumably for detecting food through vibrations generated by the wind on the surface of the sand [25]. As a defense against predators, the red flour beetle, *Tribolium castaneum*

(Tenebrionidae), displays tonic immobility (death-feigning) in response to vibrations [15, 28]. In Cydnidae and Reduviidae, individual larvae in the same colony vibrate simultaneously as a collective defense against predators [4]. The pea aphid, *Acyrthosiphon pisum* (Aphididae), drop off the host plant in response to vibrations and the humid breath of mammalian herbivores [9].

6.1.3 Vibrational Senses

The sense organs involved with vibrations are internal mechanoreceptors, called chordotonal organs, which are located in the legs and other body parts in insects [8, 12]. Two chordotonal organs in the legs—the femoral chordotonal organs and subgenual organs—are associated with vibrational reception [8]. Vibrations induce freezing responses in the Japanese pine sawyer beetle, *Monochamus alternatus* (Cerambycidae), and other longicorn beetles [35, 37, 38]. Ablation experiments on the femoral chordotonal organs in *M. alternates* were found to mediate the freezing responses, which seemed to serve as recognition of approaching predators or conspecifics [35] (Fig. 6.1).

The chordotonal organs consist of several sensory neurons and attachment cells; for example, there are 74–82 sensory neurons in *M. alternatus* and the oak longicorn beetle, *Moechotypa diphysis* (Cerambycidae) (Fig. 6.1) [35, 37]. The sensory neurons respond to vibrations via the attachment cells [8]. The femoral chordotonal organ of *M. alternatus* is attached to the tibia via a cuticular apodeme, whereas that of the brown-winged green bug, *Plautia stali*, is attached to the tibia via attachment cells, without the apodeme. In both species, vibrations are transmitted from substrates via the tibia to the femoral chordotonal organs. There are subgenual organs in the tibia of *P. stali* that lack air sacs for the transmission of vibrations in orthopteran insects [8, 32]. In *P. stali*, the sensory neurons from both chordotonal organs display electrophysiological responses to vibrations of 50–200 Hz [74]. Coleopteran insects, including *M. alternatus* and *M. diphysis*, do not have subgenual organs [35, 37]. Other external mechanoreceptors can detect strain on cuticular surfaces [4, 14].

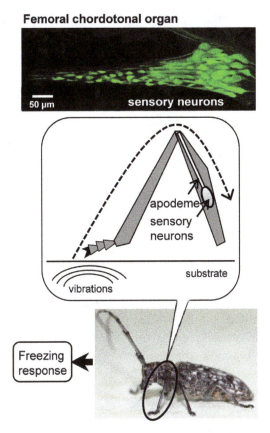

Figure 6.1 Femoral chordotonal organs of *Monochamus alternatus* mediate freezing responses to vibrations. Vibrations are transmitted from substrates, via the tibia and a cuticular apodeme, to the femoral chordotonal organs, which include sensory neurons. Modified from Takanashi et al. [35].

6.1.4 Application of Vibrations in Plant Protection

The importance of physical pest control for plant protection has increased in response to societal needs for environmentally friendly alternatives to synthetic pesticides [23, 33, 40]. Knowledge of the sensitivities and behaviors in response to vibrations is applicable to pest control for behavioral manipulation and disruption. Vibration exciters and the temporal and spectral characteristics of the vibrations are essential for the application of artificial vibrations to insect pests. Below, we present some detailed examples of the disruption of (i) vibrational communication or (ii) behavior other than communication.

It is a rational strategy to disrupt vibrational communication between sexes with artificial vibrations in pest species that exert vibrational communication. In the American grapevine leafhopper, *Scaphoideus titanus* (Cicadellidae), a vector of the lethal grapevine disease, the males produce disturbance vibrations against other males as well as sexual signals to attract females [27]. Eriksson et al. [7] demonstrated that an electromagnetic shaker could be used to mimic disturbance vibrations in field tests with *Scaphoideus titanus*, thereby simulating artificial mating disruption. The vibrational amplitude threshold for efficacy in mating disruption was validated in a field of grapevines [24]. Other examples of communication disruption have been described in psyllid species (e.g., Lujo et al. [26] for *Diaphorina citri* and Avosani et al. [1] for *Bactericera cockerelli*).

In Cerambycidae and other coleopteran families, a series of behaviors is displayed in response to vibrations (Table 6.1). However, vibrational communication for mate location has not yet been observed in longicorn beetles [2, 35, 38]. These results indicate that artificial vibrations can disrupt an assortment of behaviors other than sexual communication for pest control. *Monochamus alternatus*, the vector of pine wilt disease [18, 42], demonstrates freezing and startle responses when exposed to vibrations below 1 kHz [35]. Furthermore, vibrations of 60 and 120 Hz induce tonic immobility and startle responses in adults of the sap beetle, *Phenolia (Lasiodites) picta* (Nitidulidae), which infests rotten fruits of the Japanese apricot [17]. Because freezing and tonic immobility involve the cessation of locomotion and other behaviors, low-frequency vibrations are assumed to disrupt feeding, oviposition, and residence on host plants. Preliminary experiments have shown that feeding and other behaviors in *M. alternatus* are disrupted by low-frequency vibrations (Takanashi et al. unpublished data). Additionally, vibrations heightened escape responses from the host plant in *P. (L.) picta* larvae [16]. Therefore, low-frequency vibrations might be useful for pest control in longicorn and other beetles.

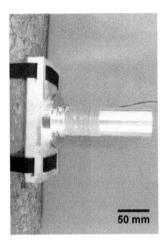

Figure 6.2 A vibration exciter made using giant magnetostrictive materials. The exciter is attached to the tree horizontally to induce behavioral responses from insects. Adapted from Takanashi et al. [36].

On the basis of our findings on vibrational sensitivity in longicorn and other beetles, we are currently developing a new technological device for pest control using artificial vibrations. We created a prototype of a vibration exciter using a giant magnetostrictive material to generate vibrations at large amplitudes on trees (Fig. 6.2). This giant magnetostrictive material is an alloy composed of iron and rare metals that exhibits a large magnetostrain, that is, a strain caused by a magnetic field [34]. This exciter generates vibrations that are expected to manifest enough low-frequency amplitudes to disrupt the behaviors of pests [35]. Additionally, the intermittent application of pulsed vibrations can decrease the possibility of vibration habituation [17]. Our pilot experiments with the giant magnetostrictive material vibration exciter attached to a tree demonstrated the disruption of behavior in *M. alternatus* (H. Sakamoto, T. Koike, N. Fukaya, T. Takanashi, unpublished data) and *P. stali* [39]. Future studies are required to thoroughly explore and resolve several issues, including the installation of the exciter for efficient vibrational transmission and the possibility of side effects on plants and nontarget beneficial insects [23, 36]. Such new pest control technologies can help in reducing the need to apply synthetic pesticides and can become part of integrated pest management in conjunction with other physical technologies [33, 40] in a variety of insects.

6.2 Contribution of Soybean Leaf Trichomes to the Resistance of *Spodoptera Litura*

6.2.1 Background

Morphological factors are important for pest resistance in plants. In the soybean plant, leaf trichomes of PI 227687 and others have been shown to contribute to herbivore resistance [43, 44]. The soybean variety Himeshirazu, which has a strong resistance to the major soybean pest *Spodoptera litura* (Lepidoptera: Noctuidae) larvae, has many trichomes on the leaf surface, and it is well known that trichomes contribute to the resistance. Similarly, the variety IAC100 also possesses well-developed trichomes on the leaf surface, and the trichomes prevent young *S. litura* larvae from walking on the leaves when the larvae attack the plant. New research has been conducted to investigate the relationship between the chemical and physical properties of the leaf trichomes in terms of their resistance to *S. litura* larvae. The soybean varieties used in this study were Enrei (or Tamahomare or Hougyoku) (nonresistant) and Himeshirazu and IAC100 (resistant to *S. litura* larvae).

6.2.2 Preference Change with and without Soybean Leaf Trichomes

Using the method of Hajika et al. in this study, we examined the effects of leaf trichomes in Himeshirazu and IAC100 by comparing the preferences of *S. litura* larvae [45]. In this method, two small pieces of leaves of a standard sample and a test sample were placed in respective Petri dishes, and a third instar *S. litura* larva was introduced into each Petri dish. Our observations evaluated the degree of feeding damage to both samples after a particular amount of time (11 points, scale from 0 to 10). S is the amount of feeding damage for the standard varieties, and T is the amount of feeding damage for the test varieties.

$$C = 2 \times \frac{\sum T}{\sum S + \sum T}.$$

The C value was a number between 0 and 2. If the preference for the test variety was lower than that for the standard variety, the value was less than 1. If the preference for the test variety was higher than that for the standard variety, the value was more than 1.

Using this method, (1) we conducted experiments using Enrei as the standard variety and Himeshirazu or IAC100 as the test varieties. The resulting C values were 0.184 and 0.194, respectively, with both showing low preferences. Then, (2) we conducted experiments using Enrei as the standard variety and Himeshirazu or IAC100, with their trichomes removed with razor blades, as the test varieties. The results showed that the C values were 0.284 and 0.315, respectively. The numbers of the C values were higher than 0.184 and 0.194. Additionally, (3) Himeshirazu or IAC100 were used as the standard varieties, and Himeshirazu or IAC100, with removed trichomes, were used as test varieties. The resulting C values were 1.249 and 1.303, respectively. These results indicated that the trichomes of Himeshirazu and IAC100 inhibited *S. litura* larvae feeding behaviors. The C values of each are summarized in Table 6.2.

Table 6.2 The C values in each experiment

	Standard variety (S)	Test variety (T)	Number of repetitions	C value[a]
(1)	Enrei	Himeshirazu	12	0.184
	Enrei	IAC100	12	0.194
(2)	Enrei	Himeshirazu (trichomes removed)	24	0.284
	Enrei	IAC100 (trichomes removed)	24	0.315
(3)	Himeshirazu	Himeshirazu (trichomes removed)	42	1.249
	IAC100	IAC100 (trichomes removed)	30	1.303

[a]$C = 2ST/(SS+ST)$.

6.2.3 Chemical Analysis of Trichome Components

The authors discovered that when *S. litura* larvae feed upon the Himeshirazu and IAC100 varieties (resistant to *S. litura*) and the Enrei or Tamahomare (nonresistant) varieties, isoflavones such as daidzein and formononetin accumulated in the damaged leaves [46]. Their chemical structures are shown in Fig. 6.3.

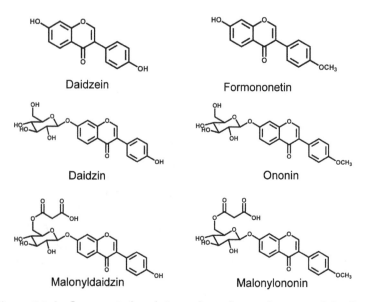

Figure 6.3 Isoflavones induced in soybean leaves because of feeding damage from *Spodoptera litura* larvae.

To investigate the localization of daidzein and formononetin biosynthesized on soybean leaves (variety: Tamahomare), the iMScope *TRIO* microscope (Shimadzu, Kyoto, Japan) was used to obtain MS imaging data. Using the soybean leaves damaged by *S. litura* larvae, the periphery of the treated area was excised and then was analyzed on the iMScope *TRIO*. As a result, MS images showed that both substances were detected in the trichomes (Fig. 6.4). As mentioned above, Tamahomare does not show any resistance to *S. litura* larvae. Currently, we are analyzing the components induced in the trichome as a result of feeding damage using the resistant varieties Himeshirazu and IAC100.

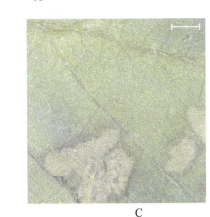
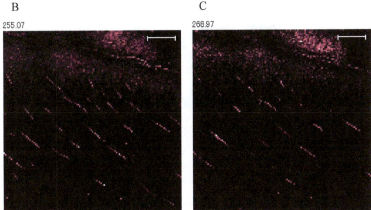

Figure 6.4 MS imaging of Tamahomare leaves damaged by *Spodoptera litura*. Optical image (A) Daidzein, (B) Formononetin, and (C) Streaky MS image matched the trichome.

6.2.4 Observation and Measurement of Trichome Physical Parameters

Alternatively, on the basis of our morphological observations and sense of touching on the leaves, it was expected that the resistant varieties Himeshirazu and IAC100 have characteristic traits on the trichomes. In this study, we measured the lengths and angles of four species of trichomes (Himeshirazu, IAC100, Tamahomare, and Hougyoku) using an OLS41003D measurement laser microscope (Olympus, Tokyo, Japan). The trichomes of Himeshirazu and IAC100 (both resistant) tended to be longer than those of Tamahomare and Hougyoku (both nonresistant) (Fig. 6.5A). Moreover, the angles of the trichomes of Himeshirazu and IAC100 were larger than those of Tamahomare and Hougyoku (Fig. 6.5B). The cross-sections of all trichomes were close to a perfect circle, and the trichomes of Himeshirazu and IAC100 were thinner than those of the nonresistant varieties (data not shown).

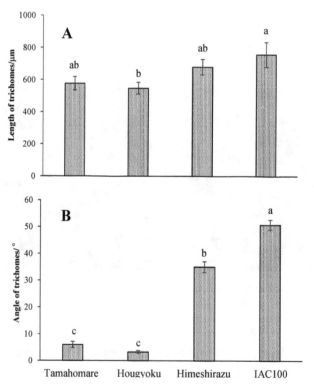

Figure 6.5 Trichome lengths (A) and angles (B) for each variety. Different letters indicate significant differences. (n = 12~15, Mean ± SEM, Tukey–Kramer's HSD test, $p < 0.05$).

6.2.5 Discussion

Hajika et al. showed that *S. litura* larvae had a weak feeding preference for Himeshirazu using a simple test method [45], and we confirmed their weak preference for IAC100. Furthermore, we discovered that the C values were higher than those of both species without trichomes. These results suggested that the trichomes of resistant varieties played an important role in weak larval feeding preference. In other words, we conclude that some trichome traits influenced larval feeding behaviors. One possible reason for this phenomenon could be the presence of chemicals in or on the surface of trichomes. For example, it is well known that the sticky secretions from trichomes (glandular hairs) deter pest movements. This phenomenon has been reported in *Lactuca sativa* (Asteraceae) [47], *Solanum polyadenium* and *S. berthaultii* (Solanaceae) [48–50], and the genus of tomatoes (*Lycopersicon*) [51]. Sticky secretions are either constantly produced or produced during herbivore attacks. Glandular hairs are different forms of soybean trichomes. When their trichomes were removed, however, the C values increased, as shown in Table 6.2. These results might suggest that some chemicals that are accumulated in trichomes play an important role in the defense against *S. litura* herbivory in Himeshirazu and IAC100.

The characteristics of trichomes in soybean leaves have been mainly focused on their density and length [52–57]. The numbers of trichomes per soybean leaf are controlled by a single gene [55] and are determined early in leaf growth [58]. In other words, the younger the leaves were, the denser the trichomes observed. If young leaves are severely damaged, it would be impossible for soybean plants to grow continuously. Considering the function(s) of trichomes, this strategy is reasonable to reduce larval performance. In fact, the upper leaves display stronger resistance [53]. Presently, no clear relationships have been shown between the physical properties of trichomes and defensive traits in Himeshirazu and IAC100.

One of the authors is interested in determining which chemicals are responsible for trichome hardness. Although the structure of the cell wall depends on polysaccharide composition, there are reports of large amounts of silicon in the trichome [59]. Silicon accumulates in plants as silicates and contributes to leaf hardness, which is called the plant opal. It is mainly found in Poaceae but has recently been found in mulberry leaves [60].

We would like to identify the chemical factors that enhance the hardness of trichomes.

More investigations are required to reveal the relationship between chemicals and the physical properties of the leaf trichomes in terms of the resistance varsities Himeshirazu and IAC100 against *S. litura* larval herbivory.

6.3 Insect Pheromone Communication

6.3.1 Background

Insects communicate with each other via the release of volatile chemicals and their reception. A typical example is the chemical communication via sex pheromone in moths, which is used for individual recognition between males and females. Female moths *de novo* biosynthesize species-specific sex pheromones and emit them into the atmosphere from their pheromone glands. The male moths detect the female sex pheromones; recognize the presence of conspecific female moths, triggering mating behavior; and localize to the pheromone source, which is a female moth. In 1959, sex pheromone was first discovered by Butenandt et al. in the silkworm moth, *Bombyx mori* [62]. Since then, sex pheromones have been discovered from insect species belonging to various genera and families, and their chemical structures have been determined in a large number of insect species to date (Pherobase; http://www.pherobase.com/). Generally, sex pheromones are composed of blends (pheromone blends), in which several components with different chemical structures are mixed in different proportions [73]. For example, a clearwing moth, *Nokona pernix*, uses a pheromone blend by mixing two components, (*E,Z*)-3,13-octadecadien-1-ol (E3,Z13-18:OH) and (*Z,Z*)-3,13-octadecadien-1-ol (Z3,Z13-18:OH), in a ratio of 9:1 [70]. Computer analysis of the sex pheromones of 1,572 moth species on the Pherolist website reported that more than half of the moths use pheromone blends consisting of two or more components [63]. Each moth species achieves reproductive isolation and speciation by creating a pheromone blend by mixing species-specific components in species-specific ratios. Thus, chemical

Insect Pheromone Communication | 119

communication via sex pheromones consists of the emission of the pheromone blend by females and its reception by males.

6.3.2 Reception of Pheromones

Insects use the antennae on their heads to detect various odorants in the environment. Sex pheromones are also detected with the antennae. On the antennae, there are many hair-like structures called olfactory sensilla, which contain multiple olfactory receptor neurons (ORNs). The dendrites of ORNs extend into the tip of the sensillum and express olfactory receptors (i.e., sex pheromone receptors) that receive sex pheromone components. When the olfactory receptors interact with the corresponding components, ORNs generate action potentials and transmit the signals to the glomeruli of the antennal lobe, the primary center for odor information processing in the brain. In particular, the sex pheromone information is transmitted to the macro glomerular complex (MGC), which is specialized for sex pheromone information processing in the antennal lobe. ORNs expressing the same sex pheromone receptors are projected to the same glomerulus, where the sex pheromone information is processed.

On the basis of the *Drosophila* genomic analysis, the olfactory receptors of insects were first discovered in 1999. Since then, several olfactory receptors have been identified, and their odorant selectivities have been revealed [65]. It has also been reported that insect olfactory receptors, along with the co-receptor Orco, function as ligand-gated cation channels [72] (Fig. 6.6), suggesting that they have evolved differently from mammalian olfactory receptors that function as G protein-coupled receptors (GPCRs). Sex pheromone receptor was first identified in the silkworm moth, *B. mori*, in 2004 [71]. Since then, sex pheromone receptors have been identified in more than 10 moth species to date, including the tobacco budworm moth, *Heliothis virescens*, and the adzuki bean borer moth, *Ostrinia scapulalis* [66, 68, 69]. The authors have also identified sex pheromone receptors in three moth species belonging to various families: the diamondback moth, *Plutella xylostella*, the armyworm moth, *Mythimna separata*, and the cucumber moth, *Diaphania indica* [67]. We isolated a sex pheromone receptor gene expressed in ORNs that are surrounded by support cells expressing pheromone-binding protein genes in male antennae. Functional analysis of African clawed frog, *Xenopus laevis*, oocytes identified the receptor as specifically responsive to the main component of sex pheromones in each moth. Although insect olfactory receptors typically respond to various odorants with similar chemical structures, sex pheromone receptors respond to sex pheromone components with relatively high selectivity and discriminate between them. Molecular phylogenetic analysis revealed that moth sex pheromone receptors form one cluster of insect olfactory receptors (i.e., sex pheromone receptor subfamily), suggesting that a common ancestral olfactory receptor might have evolved as sex pheromone receptors in moths [67]. Furthermore, we found that a clearwing moth, *N. pernix* (two-component pheromone blends), has two sex pheromone receptors, which belong to the sex pheromone receptor subfamily and selectively respond to the main and minor components (Mitsuno et al., unpublished data).

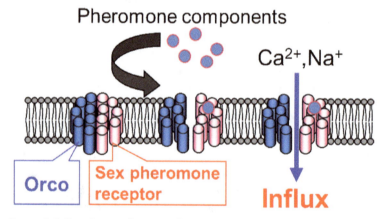

Figure 6.6 Signal transduction of insect sex pheromone receptors. The insect sex pheromone receptors, along with the olfactory receptor co-receptor (Orco), function as a ligand-gated cation channel. When sex pheromone molecules bind to the receptor, cations such as calcium and sodium nonselectively flow into the ORNs.

Now, how do moths use these multiple sex pheromone receptors to discriminate between pheromone blends with mixing species-specific components in species-specific ratios? A definitive answer to this question is elusive. However, since a male moth has multiple species-specific sex pheromone receptors and discriminates pheromone blends using the antennae with these receptors, the antennae must have a mechanism for detecting and discriminating between conspecific pheromone blends. Baker et al. reported that the proportion of olfactory sensilla that is receptive to the components of sex pheromone blends in each moth species is related to the pheromone composition [61]. Interestingly, the authors also investigated the expression patterns of the sex pheromone receptor for the main component in the antennae of each moth species, suggesting that the proportion of olfactory receptor cells expressing the primary component receptor tends to be similar to the proportion of the main component of the pheromone blend (Mitsuno et al. [67]; Mitsuno et al., unpublished data). In the future, it is expected that the elucidation of the pheromone reception mechanism of moths, which detects the compositional components of pheromone blends as well as their proportions, will lead to new sensing technologies such as the detection of gases with mixing multiple components in different proportions.

Acknowledgments

This study was partly supported by a Grant-in-Aid for Scientific Research (18KT0042 to NM, TT, and HM), grants from the Project of Bio-oriented Technology Research Advancement Institution, National Agriculture and Food Research Organization (Research Program on the Development of Innovative Technology: 02006A to TT), and Adaptable and Seamless Technology Transfer Program through Target-driven R&D from the Japan Science and Technology Agency to TT.

References

1. Avosani S., Sullivan T. E., Ciolli M., Mazzoni V., Suckling D.M. (2020). Can vibrational playbacks disrupt mating or influence other relevant behaviours in *Bactericera cockerelli* (Triozidae: Hemiptera)? *Insects*, **11**: 299.

2. Breidbach O. (1986). Studies on the stridulation of *Hylotrupes bajulus* (L.) (Cerambycidae, Coleoptera): communication through support

vibration—morphology and mechanics of the signal. *Behavioural Processes*, **12**: 169–186.

3. Čokl A., Virant-Doberlet M., Stritih N. (2000). The structure and function of songs emitted by southern green stink bugs from Brazil, Florida, Italy and Slovenia. *Physiological Entomology*, **25**: 196–205.

4. Čokl A., Virant-Doberlet M. (2003). Communication with substrate-borne signals in small plant-dwelling insects. *Annual Review of Entomology.* **48**: 29–50.

5. Endo J., Numata H. (2017). Effects of embryonic responses to clutch mates on egg hatching patterns of Pentatomidae (Heteroptera). *Physiological Entomology*, **42**: 412–417.

6. Endo J., Takanashi T., Mukai H., Numata H. (2019). Egg-cracking vibration as a cue for stink bug siblings to synchronize hatching. *Current Biology*, **29**: 143–148.

7. Eriksson A., Anfora G., Lucchi A., Lanzo F., Virant-Doberlet M., Mazzoni V. (2012). Exploitation of insect vibrational signals reveals a new method of pest management. *PloS One*, **7**: e32954.

8. Field L. H., Matheson T. (1998). Chordotonal organs in insects. *Advances in Insect Physiology*, **27**: 1–228.

9. Gish M., Dafni A., Inbar M. (2012). Young aphids avoid erroneous dropping when evading mammalian herbivores by combining input from two sensory modalities. *PloS One,* **7**: e32706.

10. Goulson D., Birch M. C., Wyatt T. D. (1994). Mate location in the deathwatch beetle, *Xestobium rufovillosum* De Geer (Anobiidae): orientation to substrate vibrations. *Animal Behaviour*, **47**: 899–907.

11. Greenfield M. D. (2002). *Signalers and Receivers.* Oxford University Press, New York.

12. Hill P. S. M. (2008). *Vibrational Communication in Animals.* Harvard University Press, Cambridge.

13. Ichikawa T, Ishii S (1974). Mating signal of the brown planthopper, *Nilaparvata lugens* Stål (Homoptera: Delphacidae): vibration of the substrate. *Applied Entomology and Zoology*, **9**:196–198.

14. Keil T. A. (1997). Functional morphology of insect mechanoreceptors. *Microscopy Research and Technique*, **39**: 506–531.

15. Kiyotake H., Matsumoto H., Nakayama S., Sakai M., Miyatake T., Ryuda M., Hayakawa Y. (2014). Gain of long tonic immobility behavioral trait causes the red flour beetle to reduce anti-stress capacity. *Journal of Insect Physiology*, **60**: 92–97.

16. Kishi M., Takanashi T. (2019a). Tonic immobility and startle responses induced by substrate-borne vibrations in the sap beetle, *Phenolia (Lasiodites) picta* (Coleoptera: Nitidulidae). *Japanese Journal of Applied Entomology and Zoology*, **63**: 13–16 (In Japanese with English abstract).

17. Kishi M., Takanashi T. (2019b). Escape behavior induced by substrate-borne vibrations in larvae of the sap beetle, *Phenolia (Lasiodites) picta* (Coleoptera: Nitidulidae). *Japanese Journal of Applied Entomology and Zoology*, **63**: 150–154 (In Japanese with English abstract).

18. Kobayashi F., Yamane A., Ikeda T. (1984). The Japanese pine sawyer beetle as the vector of pine wilt disease. *Annual Review of Entomology*, **29**: 115–135.

19. Kojima W., Ishikawa Y., Takanashi T. (2012a). Deceptive vibratory communication: pupae of a beetle exploit the freeze response of larvae to protect themselves. *Biology Letters*, **8**: 717–720.

20. Kojima W., Ishikawa Y., Takanashi T. (2012b). Pupal vibratory signals of a group-living beetle that deter larvae: are they mimics of predator cue? *Communicative and Integrative Biology*, **5**: 262–264.

21. Kojima W., Takanashi T., Ishikawa Y. (2012c). Vibratory communication in the soil: pupal signals deter larval intrusion in a group-living beetle *Trypoxylus dichotoma*. *Behavioral Ecology and Sociobiology*, **66**: 171–179.

22. Kon M., Oe A., Numata H., Hidaka T. (1988). Comparison of the mating behavior between two sympatric species *Nezara antennata* and *N. viridula* (Heteroptera: Pentatomidae) with special reference to sound emission. *Journal of Ethology*, **6**: 91–98.

23. Polajnar J., Eriksson A., Lucchi A., Anfora G., Virant-Doberlet M., Mazzoni V. (2015). Manipulating behaviour with substrate-borne vibrations—potential for insect pest control. *Pest Management Science*, **71**: 15–23.

24. Polajnar J., Eriksson A., Virant-Doberlet M., Mazzoni V. (2016). Mating disruption of a grapevine pest using mechanical vibrations: from laboratory to the field. *Journal of Pest Science*, **89**: 909–921.

25. Hanrahan S. A., Kirchner W. H. (1994). Acoustic orientation and communication in desert tenebrionid beetles in sand dunes. *Ethology*, **97**: 26–32.

26. Lujo S., Hartman E., Norton K., Pregmon E., Rohde B., Mankin R. W. (2016). Disrupting mating behavior of *Diaphorina citri* (Liviidae). *Journal of Economic Entomology*, **109**: 2373–2379.

27. Mazzoni V., Presern J., Lucchi A., Virant-Doberlet M. (2009). Reproductive strategy of the Nearctic leafhopper Scaphoideus titanus Ball (Hemiptera: Cicadellidae). *Bulletin of Entomological Research*, **99**: 401–413.

28. Miyatake T., Katayama K., Takeda Y., Nakashima A., Sugita A., Mizumoto M. (2004). Is death-feigning adaptive? Heritable variation in fitness difference of death-feigning behavior. *Proceedings of the Royal Society B: Biological Sciences*, **271**: 2293–2296.

29. Mukai H., Hironaka M., Tojo S., Nomakuchi S. (2012). Maternal vibration induces synchronous hatching in a subsocial burrower bug. *Animal Behaviour*, **84**: 1443–1448.

30. Mukai H., Hironaka M., Tojo S., Nomakuchi S. (2014). Maternal vibration: an important cue for embryo hatching in a subsocial shield bug. *PloS One*, **9**: e87932.

31. Mukai H., Hironaka M., Tojo S., Nomakuchi S. (2018). Maternal hatching synchronization in a subsocial burrower bug mitigates the risk of future sibling cannibalism. *Ecology and Evolution*, **8**: 3376–3381.

32. Nishino H., Mukai H., Takanashi T. (2016). Chordotonal organs in hemipteran insects: unique peripheral structures but conserved central organization revealed by comparative neuroanatomy. *Cell and Tissue Research*, **366**: 549–572.

33. Shimoda M., Honda K. (2013). Insect reactions to light and its applications to pest management. *Applied Entomology and Zoology*, **48**: 413–421.

34. Söderberg O., Sozinov A., Lindroos V. K. (2005). Giant magnetostrictive materials, in *Encyclopedia of Materials: Science and Technology* (Buschow K. H. J., Cahn R. W., Flemings M. C., Ilschner B., Kramer E. J., Mahajan S., Veyssière P., eds), Elsevier, Amsterdam, pp 1–3.

35. Takanashi T., Fukaya M., Nakamuta K., Skals N., Nishino H. (2016). Substrate vibrations mediate behavioral responses via femoral chordotonal organs in a cerambycid beetle. *Zoological Letters*, **2**: 18.

36. Takanashi T., Uechi N., Tatsuta H. (2019). Vibrations in hemipteran and coleopteran insects: behaviors and application in pest management. *Applied Entomology and Zoology*, **54**: 21–29.

37. Takanashi T., Nishino H. (2022). Exploitation of vibration sensing for pest management in longicorn beetles, in *Biotremology: Physiology, Ecology, and Evolution* (Hill P. S. M., Mazzoni V., Stritih Peljhan N., Virant-Doberlet M., Wessel A., eds) Springer Nature, Berlin, Germany. (in press).

38. Tsubaki R., Hosoda N., Kitajima H., Takanashi T. (2014). Substrate-borne vibrations induce behavioral responses of a leaf-dwelling cerambycid *Paraglenea fortunei*. *Zoological Science*, **31**: 789–794.

39. Uechi N., Takanashi T. (2021). Behavioral control of *Plautia stali* (Hemiptera: Pentatomidae) using vibrations, and its application in pest management. *Japanese Journal of Applied Entomology and Zoology*, **65**: 13–20 (In Japanese with English abstract).

40. Vincent C., Weintraub P., Hallman G. (2009). Physical control of insect pests, in *Encyclopedia of Insects*, 2nd ed. (Resh V. H., Cardé R. T. eds). Academic Press, Cambridge, MA, pp. 794–798.

41. Virant-Doberlet M., Čokl A. (2004). Vibrational communication in insects. *Neotropical Entomology*, **33**: 121–134.

42. Yazaki K., Takanashi T., Kanzaki K., Komatsu M., Levia D., Kabeya D., Tobita H., Kitao M., Ishida A. (2018). Pine wilt disease causes cavitation around the resin canals and irrecoverable xylem conduit dysfunction. *Journal of Experimental Botany*, **69**: 589–602.

43. Chiang H. S., Norris D. M. (1983). Morphological and physiological parameters of soybean resistance to agromyzid bean-flies. *Environmental Entomology*, **12**: 260–265.

44. Chiang H. S., Norris D. M. (1985). Expression and stability of soybean resistance to agromyzidb beanflies. *Insect Science and Its Application*, **6**: 265–270.

45. Hajika, M., Nakazawa Y., Igita K. (1993) The simple and rapid test for non-preference of *Spodoptera litura* F. (Lepidoptera: Noctuidae) to soybean [Glycine max]. *Kyushu Agricultural Research* (Japan), **55**: 40–40 (In Japanese).

46. Murakami S., Nakata R., Aboshi T., Yoshinaga N., Teraishi M., Okumoto Y., Ishihara A., Morisaka H., Huffaker A., Schmelz E. A., Mori N. (2014). Insect-induced daidzein, formononetin and their conjugates in soybean leaves. *Metabolites*, **4**: 532–546.

47. Dussourd D. E. (1995). Entrapment of aphids and whiteflies in lettuce latex. *Annals of the Entomological Society of America*, **88**: 163–172.

48. Gibson R. W., Turner R. H. (1977). Insect-trapping hairs on potato plants. *Proceedings of the National Academy of Sciences of the United States of America*, **22**: 272–277.

49. Ryan J. D., Gregory P., Tinger W. N. (1982) Phenolic oxidase activities in glandular trichomes of *Solanum berthaultii*. *Phytochemistry*, **21**: 1885–1887.

50. Tingey W. M., Gibson R. W. (1978). Feeding and mobility of the potato leafhopper impaired by glandular trichomes of *Solanum berthaultii* and *S. polyadenium*. *Journal of Economic Entomology*, **71**: 856–858.

51. Simmons A. T., Gurr G. M. 2005. Trichomes of *Lycopersicon* species and their hybrids: effects on pests and natural enemies. *Agricultural and Forest Entomology*, **7**: 265–276.

52. Broersma D. B., Bernard R. L., Luckman W. H. (1972). Some effects of soybean pubescence on populations of the potato leafhopper. *Journal of Economic Entomology*, **65**: 78–82.

53. Khan Z. R., ward J. T., Norris D. M. (1986). Role of trichomes in soybean resistance to cabbage looper, *Trichoplusia ni*. *Entomologia Experimentalis et Applicata*, **42**: 109–117.

54. Lam W. F., Pedigo L. P. (2001). Effect of trichome density on soybean pod feeding by adult bean leaf beetles (Coleoptera: Chrysomelidae). *Journal of Economic Entomology*, **94**: 1459–1463.

55. Singh B. B., Hadley H. H., Bernard R. L. (1971). Morphology of pubescence in soybeans and its relationship to plant vigor. *Crop Science*, **11**: 13–16.

56. Turnipseed S. G. (1977). Influence of trichome variations on populations of small phytophagous insects in soybean. *Environ. Entomol.* **6**: 815–817.

57. van Duyn J. W., Turnipseed S. G., Maxwell H. D. (1972). Resistance in soybeans to the Mexican bean beetle. II. Reaction of the beetle to resistant plants. *Crop Science*, **12**: 561–562.

58. Esau K. (1953). *Plant Anatomy*. John Wiley & Sons, Inc., New York.

59. Dahlin R. M., Brick M. A., Dgg J. B. (1992). Characterization and density of trichomes on three common bean cultivars. *Economic Botany*, **46**: 299–304.

60. Tsutsui O., Sakamoto R., Obayashi M., Yamakawa S., Handa T., Nishio-Hamane D., Matsuda I. (2016). Light and SEM observation of opal phytoliths in the mulberry leaf. *Flora*, **218**: 44–50.

61. Baker T. C., Domingue M. J., Myrick A. J. (2012). Working range of stimulus flux transduction determines dendrite size and relative number of pheromone component receptor neurons in moths. *Chemical Senses*, **37**(4): 299–313.

62. Butenandt V. A., Beckmann R., Stamm D., Hecker E. (1959). Uber den sexsuallockstoff des seidenspinners Bombyx mori. Reindarstellung und konstitution. *Zeitschrift für Naturforschung*, **14b**: 283–284.

63. Byers J. A. (2006). Pheromone component patterns of moth evolution revealed by computer analysis of the Pherolist. *Journal of Animal Ecology*, **75**: 399–407.

64. El-Sayed A. M. 2016. *The Pherobase: Database of Pheromones and Semiochemicals*. http://www.pherobase.com.

65. Glatz R., Bailey-Hill K. (2011). Mimicking nature's noses: from receptor deorphaning to olfactory biosensing. *Progress in Neurobiology*, **93**: 270–296.

66. Grosse-Wilde E., Gohl T., Bouche E., Breer H., Krieger J. (2007). Candidate pheromone receptors provide the basis for the response of distinct antennal neurons to pheromonal compounds. *European Journal of Neuroscience*, **25**: 2364–2373.

67. Mitsuno H., Sakurai T., Murai M., Yasuda T., Kugimiya S., Ozawa R., Toyohara H., Takabayashi J., Miyoshi H., Nishioka T. (2008). Identification of receptors of main sex-pheromone components of three Lepidopteran species. *European Journal of Neuroscience,* **28**: 893–902.

68. Miura N., Nakagawa T., Touhara K., Ishikawa Y. (2010). Broadly and narrowly tuned odorant receptors are involved in female sex pheromone reception in Ostrinia moths. *Insect Biochemistry and Molecular Biology*, **40**(1): 64–73.

69. Miura N., Nakagawa T., Tatsuki S., Touhara K., Ishikawa Y. (2009). A male-specific odorant receptor conserved through the evolution of sex pheromones in Ostrinia moth species. *International Journal of Biological Sciences,* **5**(4): 319–330.

70. Naka H., Nakazawa T., Sugie M., Yamamoto M., Horie Y., Wakasugi R., Arita Y., Sugie H., Tsuchida K., Ando T. (2006). Synthesis and characterization of 3,13- and 2,13-octadecadienyl compounds for identification of the sex pheromone secreted by a clearwing moth, Nokona pernix. *Bioscience, Biotechnology, and Biochemistry*, **70**(2): 508–516.

71. Sakurai T., Nakagawa T., Mitsuno H., Mori H., Endo Y., Tanoue S., Yasukochi Y., Touhara K., Nishioka T. (2004). Identification and functional characterization of a sex pheromone receptor in the silkmoth Bombyx mori. *Proceedings of the National Academy of Sciences of the United States of America*, **101**: 16653–16658.

72. Sato K., Pellegrino M., Nakagawa T., Nakagawa T., Vosshall L. B., Touhara K. (2008). Insect olfactory receptors are heteromeric ligand-gated ion channels. *Nature*, **452**: 1002–1006.

73. Tamaki Y., Noguchi H., Yushima T., Hirano C. (1971). Two sex pheromones of the smaller tea tortrix: isolation, identification, and synthesis. *Applied Entomology and Zoology*, **6**: 131–141.

74. Mukai H., Skals N., Takanashi T. (2020) Electrophysiological analysis of neural responses to substrate vibration in the Brown-winged green bug, *Plautia stali* (Hemiptera: Pentatomidae). *Japanese Journal of Applied Entomology and Zoology*, **64**: 1–4 (In Japanese with English abstract).

Chapter 7

Anti-Biofouling Effects against Sessile Organisms of Soft Materials

Takayuki Murosaki

Department of Chemistry, Asahikawa Medical University,
Midorigaoka-higashi 2-1-1-1, Asahikawa,
Hokkaido 078-8510, Japan

murosaki@asahikawa-med.ac.jp

Sessile organisms easily adhere to artificial submerged surfaces, and cause serious economic problems. Marine organisms have excellent strategies to protect themselves from the fouling of sessile organisms. There is few fouling on the surfaces of marine organisms (e.g. seaweeds, jellyfishes), and their bodies are composed of soft and wet materials. Recently, soft materials (hydrogels and silicone elastomers) have attention as alternative nontoxic antifouling coatings. The antifouling activities i.e. antilarval settlement and growth inhibition activities of soft materials in the laboratory and the field conditions are described.

7.1 Introduction

The sessile organisms have caused serious fouling problems by settling on the submerged artificial surfaces, e.g. ship hulls and

---

Biomimetics: Connecting Ecology and Engineering by Informatics
Edited by Akihiro Miyauchi and Masatsugu Shimomura
Copyright © 2023 Jenny Stanford Publishing Pte. Ltd.
ISBN 978-981-4968-10-2 (Hardcover), 978-1-003-27717-0 (eBook)
www.jennystanford.com

cooling water channels of the power plant [1, 2]. Tributyltin (TBT) compounds had been used widely as antifoulant until recent years. However, use of TBT-based antifouling paints on ships was banned globally, due to its high endocrine disrupting effects for marine living things (e.g. shellfish deformities and sex changes) [3]. Therefore, the development of ecofriendly antifouling technologies has been demanded. Recent studies oriented toward pollution-free paints demonstrated that the development of the nontoxic types of dissolution and self-polishing antifouling [4–7], the synthetic biodegradable antifouling compounds based on the screening of marine natural antifouling products [8–10].

In the marine environment, sessile organisms adhere on solid materials, e.g. natural rocks, woods, artificial metals and plastics, whereas soft and wet surfaces of marine living things, e. g. seaweeds, jellyfishes, and marine mammals, are not fouled by them. Inspired by this fact, the antifouling properties of soft materials (silicone elastomers and hydrogels) have been studied recently.

In this chapter, the ecology of barnacles, which are typical sessile organisms and its settlement behavior are briefly described, and then anti-biofouling activities of hydrogels in laboratory and field environments, the growth inhibition effects of soft materials against barnacles, the inhibitory effects of silicone elastomers with micro surface textures on barnacle larval settlement are discussed.

7.2 Barnacles

Barnacles are typical sessile organisms. They adhere strongly on several kinds of solid surfaces including artificial submerged materials. Thus, barnacle adhesion causes serious fouling problems in worldwide. Barnacles are crustaceans and are related to crabs and lobsters, however they spend most of their lives after settlement adhered on a substrate. So, their appearances are like shells. After settlement, adults cannot move around freely on the surface, however their larvae before settlement can swim freely and explore to find the suitable surface for the settlement.

Figure 7.1 shows the life cycle of the barnacle *Amphibalanus amphitrite*. Barnacles have two larval stages. Nauplius larvae are the earliest stage larvae of barnacles. Nauplius larvae feed phytoplankton and grow. After several days, they metamorphose into cypris larvae i.e. the settlement stage larvae. Non-feeding cypris larvae depend on limited energy reserves in their body (oil cells), and their body is designed to find and settle on a surface. Cypris larvae have a pair of antennules, of which the tops are the sense organs, at anterior inferior part of their body [11]. In pre-settlement stage, cypris larvae display the temporary attachments and explore on the surfaces with the sensory organs and determine the suitable surface for their settlement (Fig. 7.2) [12–14]. After their exploring, cypris larvae adhere firmly and permanently onto the surface by secreting the adhesive proteins [15, 16]. And then, they metamorphose into juvenile barnacles. In the post settlement stage, adult barnacles secrete the proteinaceous cement onto the substrate and broaden their adhesive area in their growth process [17].

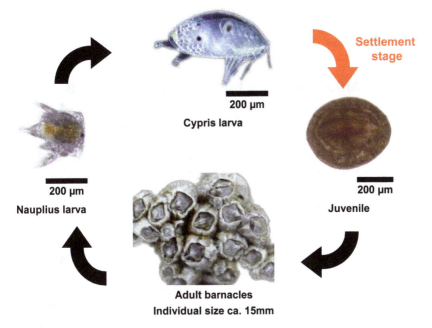

Figure 7.1 Life cycle of the barnacle *Amphibalanus amphitrite*.

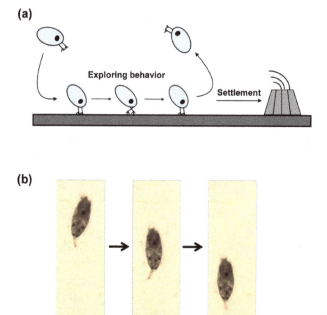

Figure 7.2 (a) Schematic illustration of exploring behavior and settlement of cypris larvae, (b) Photographs of cypris exploring behavior.

7.3 Anti-Biofouling Effects of Soft Materials

Recently, antifouling properties of soft materials (e.g. polymers, silicone elastomers, and hydrogels) have attractive attention. Some of polysaccharides (e.g. alginic acid, hyaluronic acid and pectic acid) are known to have anti-adhesive properties for cells and proteins. Furthermore, they have antifouling activities against the attachment of zoospores of *Ulva* (sea lettuce) and the settlement of cypris larvae of barnacles. On the glass surfaces, the coatings of hyaluronic acid especially showed the high antifouling activity comparing with those of alginic and pectic acids. The antifouling properties are considered to relate with the affinity of the polysaccharide with calcium in seawater [18]. On the surfaces which modified with the self-assembled monolayers (SAMs), there is no relationship between the alkyl chain length of methyl-terminated alkanethiol and the initial attachment of zoospores of *Ulva*. In contrast, the attachment of the cells of *Navicula* (diatoms) slightly increased with the reducing in the alkyl chain length [19]. Under water flow conditions, the removal rate of *Ulva* spores and *Navicula* cells from the substrates increased with the increasing in the alkyl chain length. Furthermore, the removal rates of them became approximately constant, when the friction coefficients were greater than 0.3. The results indicate that the removal activities of SAMs against *Ulva* spores and *Navicula* cells depends on primarily the friction coefficient of SAMs.

The silicone elastomers have been developed as an alternative nontoxic antifouling coating against sessile organisms. They show high release activity against sessile organisms due to their specific properties (e.g. low surface tension, low elasticity, and high smoothness) [20–23]. It was reported that the retention strength of the attached sessile organisms is minimal in the critical surface tension range between 20 and 30 mN m^{-1} [24], and the surface tension of silicone elastomer is about 20 mN m^{-1} [25].

Previously, some studies reported that the antifouling activities of hydrogels. Some polyelectrolyte-based hydrogels showed the germination inhibition effects against zoospores of seaweed [26]. Some natural polymer-based hydrogels and the poly(vinyl alcohol) (PVA) hydrogel showed antifouling activity against barnacles [27].

It was reported that barnacle settlement behaviors on the various kinds of hydrogels with different chemical composition and elasticity [28]. Figure 7.3 shows the relationship between the barnacle larval settlements and the functional groups of hydrogels. It was found that the number of barnacle larval settlements was much lower for hydrogels than solid polystyrene. Especially, hydrogels with abundant hydroxy group (–OH) on the surfaces showed high antifouling activities. On the other hand, the relatively high larval settlement was observed on the κ-carrageenan gel having with hydroxy and sulfonic acid groups. It was indicated that the antifouling effects on larval settlement seems to be reduced by coexistence of hydroxy and sulfonic groups. Additionally, the antifouling activity of hydrogels having with amino groups was relatively lower compared to other hydrogels. The percentage of dead barnacle larvae on each hydrogel was lower than 10%, indicating low toxicity of hydrogels to barnacle cypris larvae.

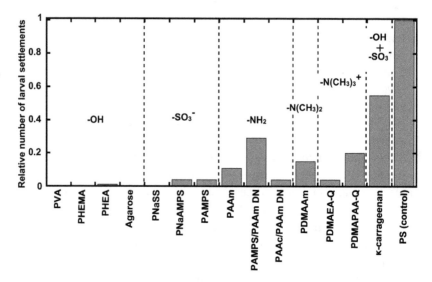

Figure 7.3 Relative number of barnacle larval settlements versus the functional groups of several hydrogels and solid polystyrene. (PVA: poly(vinyl alcohol), PHEMA: poly(2-hydroxyethylmethacrylate), PHEA: poly(2-hydroxyethylacrylate), PNaSS: poly(sodium p-styrene sulfonate), PNaAMPS: poly(2-acrylamide–2-methyl-1-propanesulfonic sodium), PAMPS: poly(2-acrylamide–2-methyl-1-propanesulfonate), PAAm: poly(acrylamide), PAAc: poly(acrylic acid), PDMAAm: poly(N,N'-dimethylacrylamide), PDMAEA-Q: poly(N,N-dimethylaminoethylacrylate, methylchloride quarternary), PDMAPAA-Q: poly (N,N-dimethylaminopropylacrylamide, methylchloride quarternary), PS: polystyrene, DN: Double-Network hydrogel).

Figure 7.4(a) shows the relationship between the barnacle larval settlements and the elasticity of hydrogels. On the hydrogels with hydroxy or sulfonic acid groups, it was found that very low larval settlements over a wide range of the elastic moduli. In contrast, the number of larval settlements increased with an increase in the elastic modulus on the hydrogels with amino acids groups. It was reported that the number of barnacle larval settlements decreased on the hydrophilic surfaces comparing with that on the hydrophobic surfaces [29]. Thus, the surface wettability might be important factor for the settlement of barnacle cypris larvae. There is a negative correlation between the elastic modulus and the swelling degrees of hydrogels (Fig. 7.4(b)). These two parameters of hydrogels cannot be changed independently. In addition, a scaling law between elasticity E and swelling degree q of hydrogels was observed experimentally in the seawater, regardless of their chemical composition. It was reported that the antifouling activity against bacterial attachment increased with the increasing in the swelling degrees of hydrogels [31], that might have the same explanation as the above results.

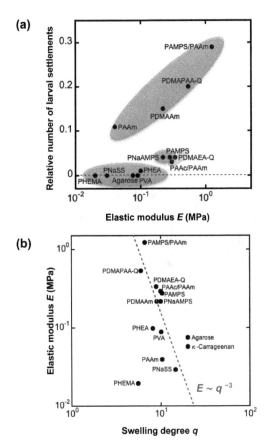

Figure 7.4 (a) Relative number of barnacle larval settlements versus the elastic modulus of several hydrogels. (b) Elastic modulus (E) versus swelling degree (q) of several hydrogels. The red dotted line shows the scaling relationship $E \sim q^{-3}$ [30].

7.4 Anti-Biofouling Effects of Hydrogels in the Ocean

As described above, soft materials are good candidates for alternative ecofriendly antifouling coatings. However, the common types of hydrogels are mechanically weak, therefore there are few reports about long-term biofouling experiments using hydrogels in the ocean. Recent studies demonstrated some mechanically tough hydrogels have a potential for use in antifouling coatings in the marine environments over long periods. It was reported that poly(2-hydroxyethyl methacrylate) (PHEMA) hydrogel coatings showed the antifouling activity against marine sessile organisms for 12-weeks [32] in the ocean. Previous report showed that metallically tough hydrogels double-network hydrogel (PAMPS/PAAm DN gel) [33] and physically crosslinked poly(vinyl alcohol) (PVA) hydrogel performed antifouling activities under the sea for 11-months [34]. Figure 7.5 shows the photographs of barnacles scraped off from the substrates after 11-months exposure under the sea. On the hydrogel surfaces, few barnacle settlements were

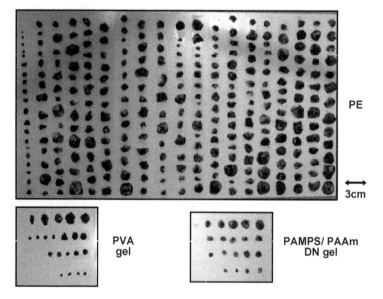

Figure 7.5 Photographs of the total quantity of settled barnacles on the solid PE, PVA hydrogel, and PAMPS/PAAm hydrogel after 330-day immersion test in the marine environment.

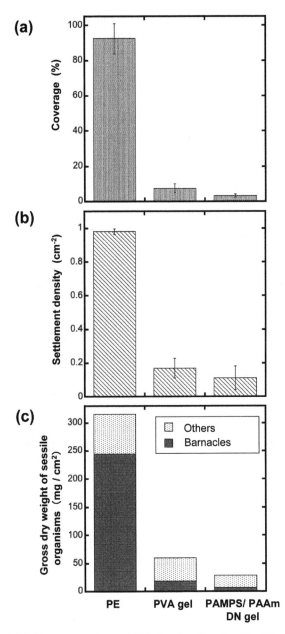

Figure 7.6 (a) The area ratio and (b) the density of settled barnacles on the solid PE, PVA hydrogel, and PAMPS/PAAm hydrogel, (c) the gross dry weight of sessile organisms after 330-day immersion test in the marine environment.

observed. In contrast, the abundance and mean size of barnacles on solid polyethylene (PE) were larger than that of hydrogels. The coverage (i.e. the percentage of barnacle adhesion area) on the submerged surfaces is shown in Fig. 7.6(a). The solid PE surface was almost entirely covered with settled barnacles (90% < coverage). In contrast, the coverage of hydrogels was less than 10%. Individual densities of settled barnacles were 0.98 cm^{-2}, 0.17 cm^{-2}, and 0.11 cm^{-2} for solid PE, PVA hydrogel and DN hydrogel, respectively as shown in Fig. 7.6(b). Figure 7.6(c) shows the dry weight of barnacles and other sessile organisms (e.g. sea squirts, sponges, and seaweeds) settled on submerged substrates. It was found that hydrogels showed high antifouling performance against the settlements of other sessile organisms in addition to the barnacle settlements.

7.5 Barnacle Growth Inhibition Effects of Soft Materials

The growth inhibition effect after the settlement of sessile organisms is also an effective antifouling technology. Previous investigations demonstrated the barnacle growth on silicone elastomers. It was reported that the morphologies of barnacle adhesive plaque bio-interface on poly(dimethylsiloxane) (PDMS) and poly(methyl methacrylate) (PMMA) [35]. On solid PMMA surface, the barnacle adhesive plaque bio-interface showed streaks and structures running from the center toward the periphery of its attachment area. In contrast, it was observed that a featureless appearance with a thick layer of a white, rubbery mass (probably primary cement) of the adhesive plaque bio-interface on soft PDMS surface. It was reported that the morphology changes of barnacle basal plates when the thickness of silicone coating was increased more than 2.0 mm [36].

Recent studies demonstrated the morphological differences of adhesive plaque bio-interface and shell appearance of barnacles grown on soft materials (PDMS and DN gel) and solid polystyrene (PS) [37, 38]. Figure 7.7 shows the photographs of basal adhesive plaque bio-interfaces and shell morphologies of barnacles grown on soft substrates (PDMS and DN gel) and solid

PS. The photographs of basal adhesive plaque bio-interfaces shows that on the solid surface (PS), the concentric and radial basal pattern was observed clearly. In contrast, an opaque basal morphology on the PDMS and a fuzzy basal pattern on the DN gel can be recognized. Furthermore, a truncated-cone shell shape with clear purple lines was observed on solid surface from the photograph of side view. In contrast, barnacles had grown with the pseudo-cylindrical shell shapes on the PDMS and the DN gel. In addition, the unclear purple lines and almost invisible lines can be recognized on the barnacle shell appetences of the PDMS and the DN gel, respectively.

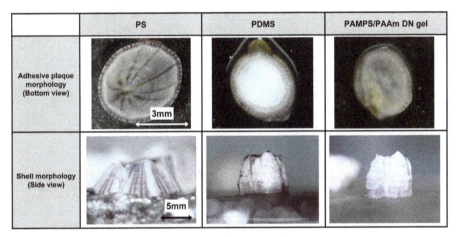

Figure 7.7 Photographs of basal adhesive plaque bio-interfaces at 70 days (above), and side views of shell morphologies at 172 days of barnacles (below) grown on various substrates.

Figure 7.8 shows the result of three-dimensional analysis of the basal plate morphology [38]. The barnacle basal plate on solid surface was almost flat (h/d ratio < 1%). In contrast, barnacles grown on the soft materials had the bell-shaped basal plates (h/d ratio = 5 ~ 13%).

A growth model of barnacles on solid materials was proposed by Saroyan et al. [39]. According to the model, the barnacle shell wall is pulled down by the muscles contraction and presses the basal edge of the shell wall tightly down on the substratum during their growing process. Thus, it is assumed that no deformation of the solid substrate and basal plate occurred on the solid surface, and the barnacle growth kept horizontally, then a truncated-cone shell shape with a flat basal plate was formed. In contrast, it is assumed that soft substrates deformed and barnacles grew vertically and a pseudo-cylindrical shell shape with a bell-shaped basal plate was formed.

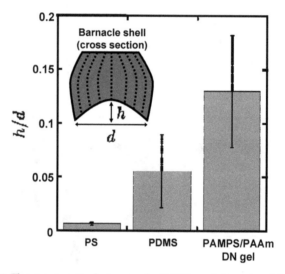

Figure 7.8 The mean ratio between depth (h) and diameter (d) of basal plates for barnacles grown on various substrates.

From the results, the barnacle shell morphology depends on the stiffness and the deformability of the substratum. The results of barnacle growth on solid PS indicate that the strong adhesion between the basal plate and solid surface by thin cement layer. On the other hand, the opaque and fuzzy basal morphologies on soft materials indicate the weak adhesion by secretion of an abundance of cement materials.

7.6 Anti-Barnacle Settlement Activity of Microstructured Silicone Elastomers

Recently, the surface microstructure modification of soft silicone elastomers for the development of antifouling technologies have been also studied. Some investigations have demonstrated that the antifouling activities of the artificial microstructures and the surfaces of marine organisms against sessile organisms. Barnacle settlements were reduced by more than 60% on microstructured silicone elastomer than that on the smooth surface [40]. The sharklet AF, which inspired by shark skin, showed the inhibition effects for the bacterial adhesion and growth [41]. It was reported that the synergistic antifouling activities of the surface micro patterning inspired by crab and surface chemical compositions [42].

Recently, it was reported that the relationship between the antifouling activity against barnacles and the surface topography of micro-pit arrays of the silicone elastomer: PDMS [43]. Figure 7.9(a) shows the SEM images of the PDMS surfaces with the 18 different types of micro-pit arrays, and the surfaces have the three characteristic geometric parameters, i.e. pore size, rim width, and depth of pits on the surfaces (Fig. 7.9(b)).

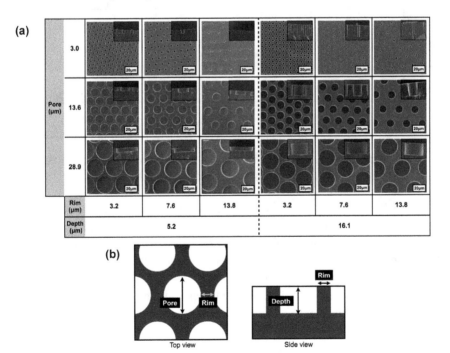

Figure 7.9 (a) The SEM images of the PDMS surfaces with the 18 different types of micro-pit arrays. Large figures show top view of the surfaces, and upper right small figures show side view of them. (b) the geometric parameters of micro-pit arrays (pore size, rim width, and depth).

Figure 7.10 shows the barnacle larval settlements on the PDMS surfaces with micro-pit arrays and the PDMS flat surface. It was found that there is no correlation between the barnacle larval settlements and the pore sizes of surface pits in the range of 3.0~28.9 μm diameter. In contrast, the larval settlements tended to decrease with an increase in the rim width and depth of the surface pits. Thus, the antifouling activities might have a correlation with the rim width and the depth of surface microstructures.

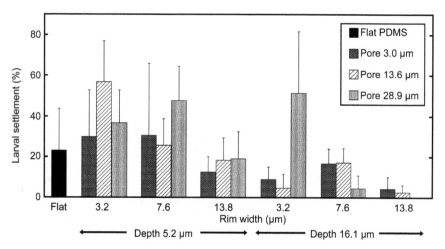

Figure 7.10 The percentage of barnacle larval settlement of the PDMS surfaces with the 18 different types of micro-pit arrays.

Figure 7.11 shows the relationship between the barnacle larval settlements and the roughness factor (r) (the ratio of true area of the surface to the projected area) of micro-pit arrays. The number of larval settlements increased with an increase in the roughness factor (r) on the surfaces with 5.2 μm of pit depth. In contrast, few larval settlements were found on the surfaces with 16.1 μm of pit depth without the dependence of roughness factor. Furthermore, the number of larval settlements was lower than that of flat PDMS surface ($r = 1$) in most surfaces with 16.1 μm of pit depth. Thus, the geometric parameter of pit depth of the PDMS surface with micro-pit arrays might be the dominant factor for the antifouling activity against the barnacle larval settlement.

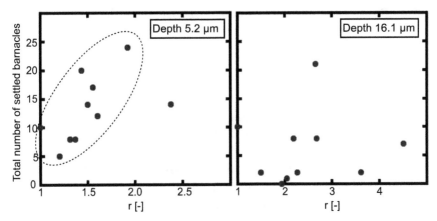

Figure 7.11 The total number of settled barnacles versus the roughness factor (r) of the PDMS surfaces with the 18 different types of micro-pit arrays.

During their exploring behavior, cypris larvae release temporary adhesive cement onto the surface [44, 45]. On the surfaces with deep pits (i.e. with large roughness factor), barnacle cypris larvae need an abundance of cement to fill the deep pits compared to the shallow pits, and obtain large surface area and establish strong adhesive cement layer. Thus, cypris larvae might inhibit to settle on the surfaces with deep pits.

7.7 Conclusion

In conclusion, soft materials, e.g. hydrogels and silicone elastomers demonstrated antifouling activities against sessile organisms in both laboratory and field conditions. The wettability as well as softness of the substrates affected the settlement of sessile organisms. Furthermore, the hydroxy functional group on the surfaces demonstrated high antifouling performance in laboratory and in ocean. In addition, soft substrates showed the growth inhibition effects against settled barnacles. Specific microstructured surface modification on silicone elastomers were useful for preventing of barnacle larval settlements. Thus, mechanically tough hydrogels with the hydroxy functional group and microstructured silicone elastomers have the potential for use in nontoxic alternative antifouling coatings in the ocean over long periods.

Acknowledgments

We gratefully acknowledge Mr. K. Hashimoto of Hashimoto Kogyou Ltd. for the supporting us to perform the field test, and Dr. Y. Nogata of Central Research Institute of Electric Power Industry for providing us with the barnacles and contributions to this work, and Prof. Y. Hirai of Chitose Institute of Science and Technology, Prof. N. Ahmed of Jagannath University, and Prof. J. P. Gong of Hokkaido University for useful discussions and contributions to this work. This research was financially supported by JSPS Grant-in-Aid for Scientific Research(B) (No. 18H01645), and Grant-in-Aid for Scientific Research(C) (No. 18K05812).

References

1. Callow, M. E., and Callow, J. E. (2002). Marine biofouling: a sticky problem. *Biologist (London, England)*, **49**, 10--14.

2. Schultz, M. P., Bendick, J. A., Holm, E. R., and Hertel, W. M. (2011). Economic impact of biofouling on a naval surface ship. *Biofouling*, **27**, 87–98.

3. International Maritime Organization (IMO). 1999. Anti-fouling systems used on ships. Resolution A. 895(21).

4. Faÿ, F., Linossier, I., Langlois, V., Renard, E., and Vallée-Réhel, K. (2006). Degradation and controlled release behavior of ε-caprolactone copolymers in biodegradable antifouling coatings. *Biomacromolecules*, **7**, 851–857.

5. Nogata, Y. (2007). New antifouling technologies: applications of barnacle settlement and metamorphosis mechanism studies. *Sessile Organisms*, **24**, 133–139.

6. Lejars, M., Margaillan, A., and Bressy, C. (2012). Fouling release coatings: a nontoxic alternative to biocidal antifouling coatings. *Chemical Reviews*, **112**, 4347–4390.

7. Carteau, D., Vallée-Réhel, K., Linossier, I., Quiniou, F., Davy, R., Compère, C., Delbury, M., et al. (2014). Development of

environmentally friendly antifouling paints using biodegradable polymer and lower toxic substances. *Progress in Organic Coatings*, **77**, 485–493.

8. Fusetani, N. (2011). Antifouling marine natural products. *Natural Product Reports*, **28**, 400–410.

9. Qian, P.-Y., Li, Z., Xu, Y., Li, Y., and Fusetani, N. (2015). Mini-review: marine natural products and their synthetic analogs as antifouling compounds: 2009–2014. *Biofouling*, **31**, 101–122.

10. Julie, G. P., and Okino, T. (2017). Anti-fouling effects of natural compounds from marine organisms. *Journal of the JIME*, **52**, 33–37.

11. Lagersson, N. C., Garm, M., and Høeg, J. T. (2003). Notes on the ultrastructure of the setae on the fourth antennulary segment of the *Balanus amphitrite* cyprid (Crustacea: Cirripedia: Thoracica). *Journal of the Marine Biological Association of the United Kingdom*, **83**, 361–365.

12. Lagersson, N. C., and Høeg, J. T. (2002). Settlement behavior and antennulary biomechanics in cypris larvae of *Balanu s amphitrite* (Crustacea: Thecostraca: Cirripedia). *Marine Biology*, **141**, 513–526.

13. Prendergast, G. S., Zurn, C. M., Bers, A. V., Head, R. M., Hansson, L. J., and Thomason, J. C. (2008). Field-based video observations of wild barnacle cyprid behaviour in response to textural and chemical settlement cues. *Biofouling*, **24**, 449–459.

14. Crisp, D. J. (1961). Territorial behaviour in barnacle settlement. *Journal of Experimental Biology*, **38**, 429–446.

15. Phang, I. Y., Aldred, N., Ling, X. Y., Huskins, J., Clare, A. S., and Vancso, G. J. (2010). Atomic force microscopy of the morphology and mechanical behaviour of barnacle cyprid footprint proteins at the nanoscale. *J. R. Soc. Interface,* **7**, 285–296.

16. Ödling, K., Albertsson, C., Russell, J. T., and Mårtensson, L. G. E. (2006). An *in vivo* study of exocytosis of cement proteins from barnacle *Balanus improvisus* (D.) cyprid larva. *Journal of Experimental Biology,* **209**, 956–964.

17. Aldred, N., and Clare, A. S. (2008). The adhesive strategies of cyprids and development of barnacle-resistant marine coatings. *Biofouling,* **24**, 351–363.

18. Cao, X., Pettit, M. E., Conlan, S., Wagner, W., Ho, A., Clare, A., Callow, J. A., Callow, M. E., Grunze, M., and Rosenhahn, A. (2009). Resistance of polysaccharide coatings to proteins, hematopoietic cells, and marine organisms. *Biomacromolecules,* **10**, 907–915.

19. Bowen, J., Pettitt, M., Kendall, K., Leggett, G., Preece, J., Callow, M. E., and Callow, J. A. (2007). The influence of surface lubricity on the adhesion of *Navicula perminuta* and *Ulva linza* to alkanethiol self-assembled monolayers. *Journal of The Royal Society Interface*, **4**, 473–477.

20. Adkins, J. D., Mera, A. E., Roe-Short, M. A., Pawlikowski, G. T., and Brady, R. F. (1996). Novel non-toxic coatings designed to resist marine fouling. *Progress in Organic Coatings*, **29**, 1–5.

21. Brady, R. F. (2001). A fracture mechanical analysis of fouling release from nontoxic antifouling coatings. *Progress in Organic Coatings*, **43**, 188–192.

22. Anderson, C., Atlar, M., Callow, M., Candries, M., Milne, A., and Townsin, R. L. (2003). The development of foul-release coatings for seagoing vessels. *Journal of Marine Design and Operations.*, **4**, 11–24.

23. Kavanagh, C. J. (2005). Observations of barnacle detachment from silicones using high-speed video. *The Journal of Adhesion*, **81**, 843–868.

24. Baier, R. E. (2006). Surface behaviour of biomaterials: the surface for biocompatibility. *J. Mater. Med.*, **17**, 1057–1062.

25. Ishii, T. (2001). *The Handbook for the Technology of Wettability. "The Wettability of Plastic Materials."* Technosystem, Inc., Tokyo, pp. 149–218.

26. Katsuyama, Y., Kurokawa, T., Kaneko, T., Gong, J. P., Osada, Y., Yotsukura, N., and Motomura, T. (2002). Inhibitory effects of hydrogels on the adhesion, germination, and development of zoospores originating from *Laminaria angustata*. *Macromolecular bioscience*, **2**, 163–169.

27. Rasmussen, K., Willemsen, P. R., and Østgaard, K. (2002). Barnacle settlement on hydrogels. *Biofouling*, **18(3)**, 177–191.

28. Murosaki, T., Noguchi, T., Kakugo, A., Putra, A., Kurokawa, T., Furukawa, H., Osada, Y., Gong, J. P., Nogata, Y., Matsumura, K., Yoshimura, E., and Fusetani, N. (2009a). Antifouling activity of synthetic polymer gels against cypris of the barnacle (*Balanus amphitrite*) in vitro. *Biofouling*, **25**, 313–320.

29. Dahlström, M., Jonsson, H., Jonsson, P., and Elwing, H. (2004). Surface wettability as a determinant in the settlement of the barnacle *Balanus improvisus* (DARWIN). *Journal of Experimental Marine Biology and Ecology*, **305**, 223–232.

30. de Gennes, P. G. (1979). *Polymer gels. "Scaling concepts in polymer physics"*. Cornell University Press, Ithaca, pp. 128–162.

31. Eshet, I., Freger, V., Kasher, R., Herzberg, M., Lei, J., and Ulbricht, M. (2011). Chemical and physical factors in design of antibiofouling polymer coatings. *Biomacromolecules*, **12**, 2681–2685.

32. Cowling, M. J., Hodgkiess, T., Parr, A. C., Smith, M. J., and Marrs, S. J. (2000). An alternative approach to antifouling based on analogues of natural processes. *The Science of the Total Environment*, **258**, 129–137.

33. Gong, J. P., Katsuyama, Y., Kurokawa, T., and Osada, Y. (2003). Double-network hydrogels with extremely high mechanical strength. *Advanced Materials*, **15**, 1155–1158.

34. Murosaki, T., Noguchi, T., Hashimoto, K., Kakugo, A., Kurokawa, T., Saito, J., Chen, Y. M., Furukawa, H., and Gong, J. P. (2009b). Antifouling properties of tough gels against barnacles in a long-term marine environment experiment. *Biofouling*, **25**, 657–666.

35. Berglin, M., and Gatenholm, P. (2003). The barnacle adhesive plaque: morphological and chemical differences as a response to substrate properties. *Colloids and Surfaces B: Biointerfaces*, **28**, 107–117.

36. Wendt, D. E., Kowalke, G. L., Kim J. S., and Singer, I. (2006). Factors that influence elastomeric coating performance: the effect of coating thickness on basal plate morphology, growth and critical removal stress of the barnacle *Balanus Amphitrite*. *Biofouling*, **22**, 1–9.

37. Ahmed, N., Murosaki, T., Kakugo, A., Kurokawa, T., Gong, J. P., and Nogata, Y. (2011). Long-term in situ observation of barnacle growth on soft substrates with different elasticity and wettability. *Soft Matter*, **7**, 7281–7290.

38. Ahmed, N., Murosaki, T., Kurokawa, T., Kakugo, A., Yashima, S., Nogata, Y., and Gong, J. P. (2014). Prolonged morphometric study of barnacles grown on soft substrata of hydrogels and elastomers. *Biofouling*, **30**, 271–279.

39. Saroyan, J. R., Lindner, E., and Dooley, C. A. (1970). Repair and reattachment in the Balanidae as related to their cementing mechanism. *The Biological Bulletin*, **139**(2), 333–350.

40. Petronis, Š., Berntsson, K., Gold, J., and Gatenholm, P. (2000). Design and microstructuring of PDMS surfaces for improved marine biofouling resistance. *Journal of Biomaterials Science, Polymer Edition*, **11**, 1051–1072.

41. Chung, K. K., Schumacher, J. F., Sampson, E. M., Burne, R. A., Antonelli, P. J., Brennan, and A. B., (2007). Impact of engineered surface microtopography on biofilm formation of *Staphylococcus aureus*. *Biointerphases*, **2**, 89–94.

42. Brzozowska, A. M., Parra-Velandia, F. J., Quintana, R., Xiaoying, Z., Lee, Serina S. C., Chin-Sing, L., Jańczewski, D., Teo, Serena L.-M., and Vancso, J. G. (2014). Biomimicking micropatterned surfaces and their effect on marine biofouling. *Langmuir*, **30**, 9165–9175.

43. Murosaki, T., Abe, K., Nogata, Y., and Hirai, Y. (2019). Barnacle settlement behaviors on microstructured surfaces with different geometric parameters. *Journal of Photopolymer Science and Technology,* **32**(2), 303–308.

44. Nott, J. A., and Foster, B. (1969). On the structure of the antennular attachment organ of the cypris larva of *Balanus balanoides* (L.). *Philosophical Transactions of the Royal Society of London. Series B, Biological Sciences*, **256**, 115–134.

45. Walker, G., and Yule, A. (1984). Temporary adhesion of the barnacle cyprid: the existence of an antennular adhesive secretion. *Journal of the Marine Biological Association of the United Kingdom*, **64**, 679–686.

Chapter 8

Biomimetic Devices by Nano/Micro Processing

Seiji Aoyagi, Masato Suzuki, Tomokazu Takahashi, and Takeshi Ito

Department of Mechanical Engineering,
Kansai University, 3-3-35 Yamate-cho,
Suita-shi, Osaka 564-8680, Japan

aoyagi@kansai-u.ac.jp

This chapter introduces the biomimetic devices currently under research and development at Kansai University. First, the three-dimensional processing technology to manufacture biomimetic devices is discussed. Then five devices are introduced: painless needle, gripper, antibacterial surface, adhesive projections, and robot hand, inspired by mosquitoes, octopuses, cicadas, geckos, and tree frogs, respectively.

8.1 Introduction

Biomimetics research is actively being pursued to develop innovative products, including magic adhesive tapes inspired by the footpads of geckos, sharkskin swimwear for reducing fluid resistance, and Shinkansen pantographs shaped like the wings of

---

Biomimetics: Connecting Ecology and Engineering by Informatics
Edited by Akihiro Miyauchi and Masatsugu Shimomura
Copyright © 2023 Jenny Stanford Publishing Pte. Ltd.
ISBN 978-981-4968-10-2 (Hardcover), 978-1-003-27717-0 (eBook)
www.jennystanford.com

an owl for reducing wind noise [1]. According to the *Financial Times*, biomimetics will add $300 billion annually to the gross domestic product of the United States in 2026 and employ 1.6 million people [2]. Animals have obtained optimal shapes and operations through evolution. Advanced functions are easily realized by scientifically mimicking those of animals.

Biological structures are created by the bottom-up assembly of microstructures, and therefore, fine-processing technologies are required to mimic them. In this paper, we first discuss the necessity of combining the MEMS (microelectromechanical systems) processing technology with the three-dimensional processing technology to create a fine-processing technology for manufacturing biomimetic devices. Then, we introduce five devices, namely, a painless needle that mimics mosquitoes, a vacuum suction gripper that mimics the acetabulum (suction cup) of octopuses, an antibacterial nanosurface that mimics the wings of cicadas, an adhesive projection that mimics the footpads of geckos, and a robot hand that mimics the fingers of forest green tree frogs.

8.2 Fusion of MEMS with Ultra-High-Precision Three-Dimensional Processing

MEMS processing, which is based on the fine processing technology for semiconductors, revolutionizes the concepts of previous mechanical processing methods to enable the creation of fine structures of the order of micrometers or nanometers. This processing method can create 2.5-dimensional structures to transfer a shape in the depth direction; however, the manufacturing of truly three-dimensional complex fine structures is difficult. On the other hand, in biomimetics research, one often encounters not only the proboscis of a mosquito [3–5], but also many other structures, which require the mimicking of complicated three-dimensional organs in which micrometer or nanometer-sized fine structures are self-assembled. We are attempting to combine the existing MEMS technology with new fine-processing technologies such as three-dimensional shaping (the processing concept of three-dimensional printers, which are a current topic of discussion), femtosecond laser processing, and nanoimprint processing to mimic biological structures.

We use the example of a fine needle that mimics the mouth organs of a mosquito (Fig. 8.1) to schematically explain the difference between MEMS processing and three-dimensional processing. MEMS processing can only fabricate a flat needle whose tip is not pointed, as observed when viewed from the side. Therefore, it is believed that a large resistance force is generated when it punctures the skin, accompanied with significant pain during puncturing. However, by three-dimensional shaping, a needle with a sharp tip in the three-dimensional sense (like the shape of a cone) can be manufactured.

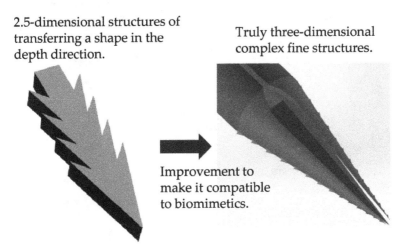

Figure 8.1 Comparison between MEMS (Micro-Electro-Mechanical Systems) fabrication (left) and three-dimensional fabrication (right): example in the microneedle mimicking a mosquito proboscis.

An ultra-high-precision laser lithographic system has been installed at Kansai University to perform three-dimensional shaping (Fig. 8.2, Photonic Professional GT, Nanoscribe, Germany). This system focuses the beam of a femtosecond laser (ultrashort pulse laser) on a microscopic region of size 200 nm (0.2 µm) in the interior of a photocurable resin to cause exposure using the two-photon absorption principle. The portions of the focused area with the required shape are exposed either by successively positioning a high-precision piezo-stage on which the sample is mounted, or by scanning and successively positioning the laser beam by reflecting it with a galvanometer mirror. Finally, by developing the exposed region, a hyper-fine structure with a resolution of 200 nm can be manufactured. Three-dimensional printers are widely used now because of reduced cost; however, only a few have the high precision required for application in biomimetics. Hence, this new device may become a useful manufacturing tool. Figure 8.3 shows a microneedle having a protrusion with a jagged edge manufactured using this system to mimic the proboscis of a mosquito [6].

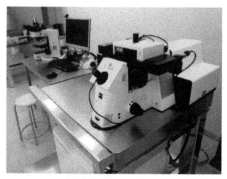
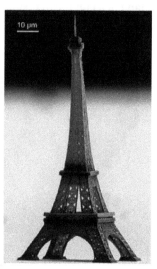

Resolution of 200 nm due to two-photon absorption principle.

Fast scanning up to 10 mm/s due to galvanometer mirror

Figure 8.2 Ultra-High-Precision three-dimensional laser lithographic system (Photonic Professional GT, Nanoscribe, Germany), which has been installed at Kansai University. Overview photograph (left) and SEM image of fabricated sample (right).

Kansai University has also introduced a device that uses a femtosecond laser beam for the fine processing of polymers, ceramics, and metals (IFRIT-D, Cyber Laser Inc.). This device has a rotating stage that can tilt with three degrees of freedom, which allows the manufacturing of three-dimensional fine structures (Fig. 8.4).

Fusion of MEMS with Ultra-High-Precision Three-Dimensional Processing | **153**

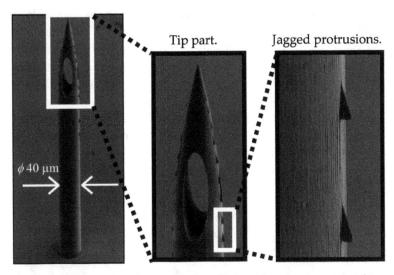

Figure 8.3 SEM images of microneedle with jagged protrusions mimicking mosquito proboscis, which was fabricated by the three-dimensional laser lithographic system.

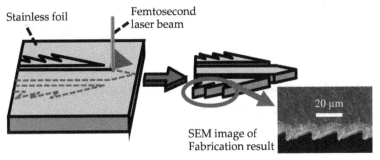

(a) Cut out the needle shape from stainless foil.

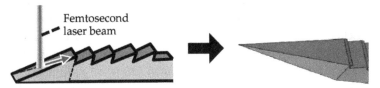

(b) Rotate by 90 degree, then process it to sharpen the tip three-dimensionally.

Figure 8.4 Three-dimensional manufacture on stainless foil by a high-power femtosecond laser beam: example of microneedle mimicking mosquito proboscis.

Such three-dimensional processing has the drawback of long processing times. Therefore, as shown in Fig. 8.5, consideration has been given to using shapes manufactured by such devices as masters, transferring them to resins by a nanoimprinting method, and using these resins as molds (negative molds) for molding resins and metals with high speed, high volume, and low cost. Kansai University has introduced an apparatus (NM0901, Meisho Kiko) that can perform both thermal nanoimprinting and UV (ultraviolet curing) nanoimprinting. In the references, we list a URL for the group of devices (a facility) that can be used at Kansai University [7].

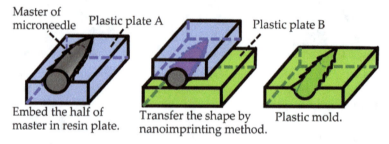

Figure 8.5 Nanoimprinting manufacture of resin mold for injecting plastic or electroforming metal on it.

8.3 Microneedles for Drawing Blood by Mimicking Mosquitoes

8.3.1 Introduction

People feel almost no pain when they are stung by mosquitoes. The development of painless needles can be accelerated by mimicking this with biomimetic methods. In terms of mechanics, a mosquito sting is less invasive and less painful because the diameter of the needle is extremely small (30 to 60 µm); hence, it is more likely to avoid the pain sites in the skin. Moreover, the needle has a unique jagged shape [8, 9], although the details of the stinging mechanism are unclear. In terms of biochemistry, the saliva of a mosquito has been reported to have an anesthetic effect [10, 11]. Among these ideas, much research has focused on the mechanical aspect and attempts were made to realize painless needles by fabricating thin needles. Hyper-fine metal needles with a diameter of 180 μm using press working have even been marketed in recent years [12].

8.3.2 Structure of the Mosquito Needle and the Stinging Motion

We have considered that, besides the thinness of the needle, the shape of the needle and the method of piercing may contribute to the reduction in the stinging pain; therefore, we observed the shape of the mosquito needle and the stinging motion of the mosquito in detail [3, 4, 13–15]. Figure 8.6 shows the scanning electron microscope (SEM) images of the needle of a mosquito photographed in our laboratory, and a schematic of the structure of the needle of the mosquito. A mosquito's proboscis is not a single needle but is composed of six organs, namely, a labrum for the path of blood, a pharynx for the path of saliva, two mandibles, and two maxillae. In addition, the proboscis fits into the sheath-shaped labium. The tips of the maxillae have protrusions with jagged edges.

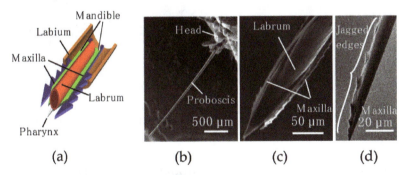

Figure 8.6 (a) Schematic structures of seven parts of mosquito proboscis, (b) SEM images of head and proboscis, (c) maxillae and labrum, and (d) magnification of maxilla.

To explain in detail the motion of the needle of the mosquito, we photographed the stinging motion using a high-speed camera and a magnifying lens with long-working distance. We verified that, while performing coordinated motions to alternately protrude the labrum and the pair of maxillae, the mosquito gradually pierces the entire needle deeper into the skin. By simulating the alternately protruding motions of the labrum and maxillae of the mosquito using the finite element method, we inferred the mechanism of the stinging motion [16, 17]. We believe that the protrusions with the jagged edge at the tips of the maxillae play a role in the following actions during stinging: (1) The skin is slashed as with the blade of a saw. (2) When the maxillae go forward, the needle is in contact with the skin only near the tip of the protrusion; hence, the contact area as well as the contact resistance reduces. (3) When the maxillae go backward, the protrusions with the jagged edge cut into the skin and become anchors to assist the forward motion of the labrum. In Fig. 8.7, we schematically show the stinging mechanism of the mosquito as inferred from the observational results obtained with the high-speed camera.

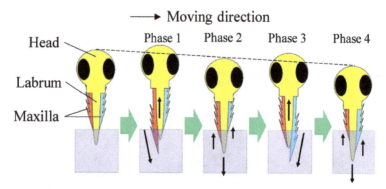

Figure 8.7 Schematic of cooperative motion of labrum and maxillae. Head and three needle parts advance downward gradually by repeating from phase 1 to phase 4 at the frequency of several Hz.

8.3.3 Manufacture of a Microneedle by Ultra-High-Precision Three-Dimensional Laser Lithography

We have used the MEMS technology to develop many minimally invasive microneedles that mimic the needle of a mosquito. Their materials range from biodegradable polymers (polylactic acid) [3] to monocrystalline silicon [4, 9] and metals [5, 18].

However, these needles cannot accurately mimic the three-dimensional shape of a mosquito proboscis; therefore, we tried to solve the problem using an ultra-high-precision three-dimensional laser lithographic method.

8.3.3.1 Manufacture of a set of three needles to mimic the labrum and two maxillae of a mosquito (faithful mimicking of the mosquito)

We manufactured a set of three fine needles that faithfully mimic the labrum and the pair of maxillae of a mosquito (Fig. 8.8). The needle that mimicked the labrum was cylindrical with an outer diameter of 30 μm and inner diameter of 20 μm, and a sharpened tip. The cross sections of the needles that mimicked the maxillae was gutter-shaped in which 1/4th was cut out from a cylinder with an outer diameter of 60 μm and inner diameter of 50 μm. We succeeded in manufacturing microneedles with a maximum length of 2 mm.

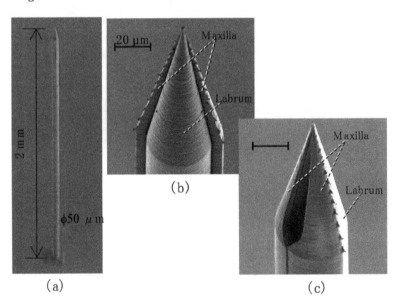

Figure 8.8 SEM image of microneedles bundling three parts imitating one labrum and two maxillae of mosquito; (a) overview, (b) back view, and (c) side view.

8.3.3.2 Proposal for needles in which two split-in-half needles are combined

The laser lithographic method has the problem of a slow processing speed; therefore, it cannot be considered an appropriate manufacturing method for blood-drawing needles, which are intended to be single-use needles. This problem can be solved by using a manufactured microneedle as a master, manufacturing a mold by plating the master to make it mold-releasing, and using the mold to obtain a polymeric needle by injection molding or a metal needle by electroforming. However, among the set of three needles, it is difficult to manufacture the mold for the hollow needle that mimics the labrum.

To solve this problem, we present a microneedle that is easy to transfer and maintains the functions of the labrum and maxillae of the mosquito [6]. Figure 8.9 shows the general shape and dimensions of the microneedle. The hollow cylindrical microneedle with a sharpened tip is halved in the longitudinal direction. The portions other than the tip have a gutter shape where a fluid can flow in the inner groove. The tip surface is given a protrusion with a jagged edge similar to that of the maxillae of the mosquito. Since the split-in-half needle unit does not have a hollow structure, it is easy to transfer the shape.

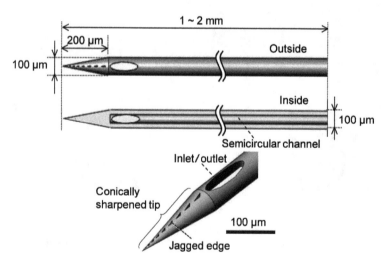

Figure 8.9 General shape and dimensions of a half-microneedle having a gutter.

Two such half-microneedles are joined together to make a hollow microneedle. It is also possible to draw in or discharge liquid through the hole that is made in the side surface. In addition, even after the two halves are joined, it is possible to operate each of the needles independently. Therefore, as shown in Fig. 8.10, it is possible to mimic the maxillae of the mosquito by alternatively moving each of the needles forward. In other words, with this microneedle, the three parts of the proboscis (one labrum and two maxillae) of the mosquito are modeled as two needles.

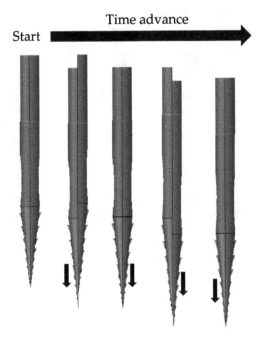

Figure 8.10 Alternative inserting motion of combined two half-microneedles.

8.3.3.3 Manufacture of split-in-half microneedles and evaluation of the piercing and blood-drawing functions

We manufactured needle shapes using a three-dimensional laser lithographic system (Nanoscribe). The SEM images are shown in Fig. 8.11. For the material, we used IP-S, which is a special photocuring resist for this device. We performed a stinging test using the hollow microneedle that combined two manufactured split-in-half needles. For the stinging target, we used an artificial skin (Young's modulus: 0.4 MPa) manufactured using PDMS (polydimethylsiloxane, a kind of silicone rubber). For the stinging motion, we tried three modes, namely, the coordinated vibration mode shown in Fig. 8.10, a vibration mode in which the two needles are vibrated in the same phase, and a mode that advances without any vibration. The vibration frequency and amplitude were 10 Hz and 0.05 mm, respectively.

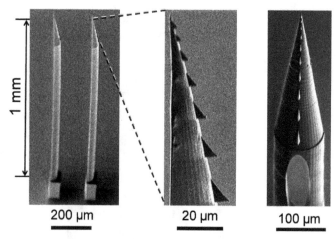

Figure 8.11 SEM images of split-in-half microneedles manufactured using a three-dimensional laser lithographic system (Nanoscribe).

We performed stinging three times for each stinging motion, and in all the cases, the microneedle pierced the artificial skin without buckling. Figure 8.12 shows the piercing resistance of the artificial skin when the microneedle pierced to a depth of 0.8 mm from the surface. We found that the piercing resistance force was the smallest in the case where the two needles pierced while cooperatively vibrating as in a mosquito.

We then inserted a hollow microneedle made by joining the two split-in-half needles into a drop of human whole blood to determine whether blood could be drawn in by the capillary action; the blood was drawn at a speed of 0.025 µL/s. We also performed a drawing-in experiment using a vacuum pump, where the speed was 0.2 µL/s, and we obtained at least 6 µL of blood. The amount of blood needed for a diabetes test is 0.3 µL; thus, it would be possible to draw blood within several seconds.

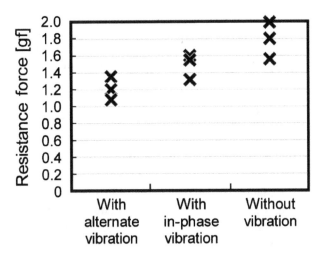

Figure 8.12 Resistance forces under three conditions when the insertion distance is 0.8 mm.

8.3.4 Manufacture of a Microneedle Using a Femtosecond Laser

The laser lithographic method requires considerable time and cost for manufacturing one needle; hence, it is not an appropriate manufacturing method for needles used for drawing blood, which are intended to be single-use needles. Therefore, it is necessary to use this as a master to be transferred to a metal or biodegradable plastic. Currently, we are engaged in the research and development of electroforming and injection molding technologies for this purpose [19]. In addition, it is possible to use manufacturing methods that directly process commercially available small-diameter pipes or foil-like plates using stainless steel as the material, which is excellent from the viewpoint of strength and biocompatibility [20]. We manufactured microneedles by femtosecond laser processing [21, 22].

8.3.4.1 Hollow needle mimicking the labrum

We manufactured a sharp, hollow microneedle by cutting the tip of a hyper-fine stainless steel pipe (Ohbakiko Co., Ltd.) of diameter 50 μm at a slant of 15°. Our evaluation standard was that the hole portion was not covered by fused stainless steel and that debris did not adhere to the cut surface. We determined the optimal conditions to be a wavelength of 390 nm (second harmonic), power of 0.3 mW, and scanning speed of 0.1 mm/s.

8.3.4.2 Plate-shaped needle having a protrusion with a jagged edge

We manufactured a microneedle with a jagged tip, mimicking the maxillae of a mosquito, by processing a stainless steel foil (Nilaco Corporation) having a thickness of 30 μm. We used a beam with a diameter of 1.2 μm to cut out from the foil a needle shape having a protrusion with a jagged edge with a tooth depth of 7 μm and pitch of 20 μm. We arranged for it to be rotated by 90° with the longitudinal direction as the axis so that the jagged shape was at the top, and then we processed it so that the tip angle was 15°. By performing laser processing in this way twice, once on the upper surface and once on the side surface, it was possible to perform three-dimensional sharpening of the needle tip.

8.3.4.3 Comparison with the proboscis of a mosquito

Figure 8.13 shows the comparison between the manufactured stainless steel microneedle and the proboscis of a mosquito. Figure 8.13(a) shows the SEM image of the proboscis of a mosquito. It is composed of a pair of maxillae and a labrum in the middle. Figure 8.13 (b) shows the schematic drawing of a microneedle that mimics the proboscis of a mosquito as manufactured in this research, and the SEM images of each of the microneedles. We can see that the labrum and maxillae are mimicked.

8.3.4.4 Performance evaluation

We performed a stinging test using the combination of a pair of stainless steel microneedles with jagged edges and a hollow microneedle. As in the case of plastic needle prepared by three-dimensional laser lithography as mentioned in the previous section, the resistance force decreased by 40% when vibration was included. Moreover, we successfully drew blood by immersing the tip of the hollow needle that mimics the central labrum in a drop of human whole blood.

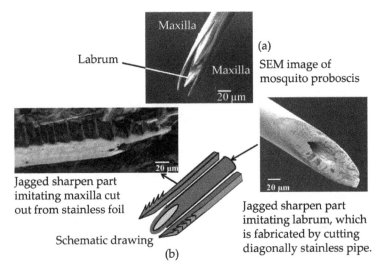

Figure 8.13 Comparison between the stainless microneedles fabricated by femtosecond laser beam and the mosquito proboscis.

8.4 Vacuum Suction Gripper That Mimics the Octopus Acetabulum

8.4.1 Introduction

Currently, in the transport and assembly of automated parts, a unique robot hand is often used for each part. There is therefore a desire for a general-purpose hand that can grip parts of various sizes and shapes.

In this research, we focused on the flexible gripping ability of an octopus to develop a gripper that mimics its acetabulum. The octopus can ingeniously move muscles that are flexible and have a large generating force to grip items such as preys using its arms and acetabula. As shown in Fig. 8.14, an acetabulum has an infundibulum and acetabular muscles [23]. First, it expands the infundibulum to adhere tightly to the target. Then, it contracts the acetabular muscles to reduce the pressure of the tightly closed space, creating suction [24]. Grippers have been reported that mimic this type of octopus suction method, and all of them deform a membrane after tightly closing in to expand the space, thereby lowering the pressure of the space according to the Boyle–Charles law [25–28]. We also developed a hand that creates suction by using the air pressure difference that is created by reducing the pressure within the gripper [29, 30].

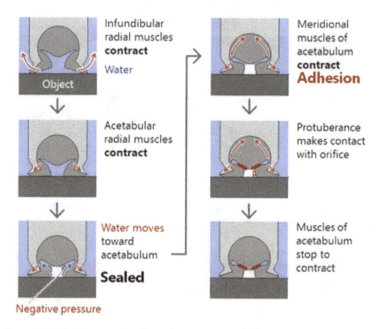

Figure 8.14 Suction mechanism of octopus acetabulum.

8.4.2 Principle and Structure

Figure 8.15 shows the principle and structure of the suction gripper. The gripper is a rubber bag that contains particles such as glass beads. The thickness of the rubber at the bottom is less than that elsewhere, and the rubber operates like the acetabulum. Around the acetabulum is a circular tube that provides a space so that a membrane can deform, and the filter at its upper edge prevents particles from entering. Since the rubber bag containing the particles is flexible, its shape changes according to the shape of the target when pressed against the target. Then, when the pressure inside the gripper is lowered, the pressure difference between inside and outside the gripper causes the rubber bag to press on the particles; hence, the rigidity of the bag increases. This phenomenon is called a jamming transition. At the same time, the membrane deforms, the pressure within the tightly closed space decreases, and suction occurs. The target can be released by supplying air into the gripper to increase the internal pressure to atmospheric pressure.

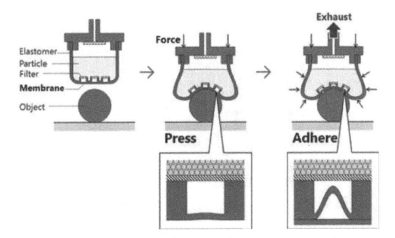

Figure 8.15 Principle and structure of the suction gripper.

8.4.3 Gripper Manufacture and Gripping Experiment

We developed the two types of acetabula shown next. In one case, the gripper has multiple acetabula arranged in a bag, and in the other case, the gripper has a single acetabulum. The manufacturing methods of both the grippers are the same. First, to manufacture the rubber portion, silicone rubber was poured into a mold, hardened, and peeled off to mold the rubber. A filter was fixed inside the rubber with an adhesive, and the rubber was filled with glass beads (diameter: 0.7 to 1.0 mm). Finally, this structure was attached to a metal jig.

8.4.3.1 Semispherical gripper with multiple acetabula

The manufactured gripper is shown in Fig. 8.16. We verified the ability of the semispherical gripper for general use. The target was aluminum with a flat, spherical, stepped, or grooved surface. We investigated the success rate for gripping these objects. Then, we similarly evaluated the effect of surface wetness. We performed the experiment twenty times. The experimental results are shown in Fig. 8.17.

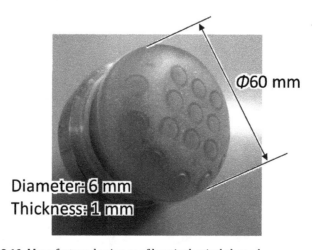

Figure 8.16 Manufactured gripper of hemispherical shaped.

In the case of a flat surface, the area ratio of the gripper and target has an influence. In general, it is easy to grip a flat plate that is larger than a gripper is, while it is difficult to grasp a small plate due to the effect of the edge portion. However, here, the area of the gripper is 2,830 mm^2, and as shown in Fig. 8.17(a), the gripping success rate is high regardless of the area of the target.

In the case of a curved surface, whether the gripper can deform by following the target is important. As shown in Fig. 8.17(b), the gripping success rate is 100% for a cylindrical tube with a radius as small as 10 mm. We believe that the gripping success rate decreased for a diameter of 5 mm because the 6-mm-diameter acetabulum could not form an adhering surface with the target.

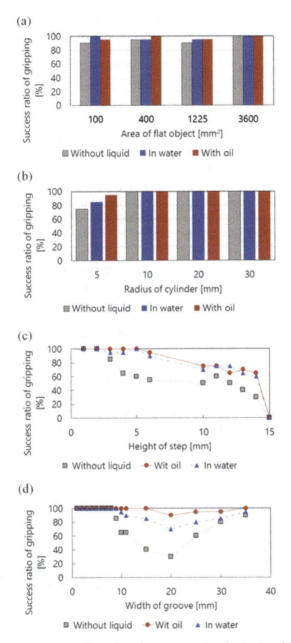

Figure 8.17 Experimental results of success ratio of gripping for several shaped objects under the condition of surface wettability.

In the case of a stepped surface, it is important for the gripper to have flexibility for sharp angles. As shown in Fig. 8.17(c), for a step height of up to 5 mm, the gripping success rate is 100%. However, thereafter, the gripper cannot tightly adhere to the target and the gripping success rate decreases. For a step height of 15 mm, the gripper cannot grip the target at all.

In the case of a groove, similar to the case of a stepped surface, the flexibility of the gripper has an influence. As shown in Fig. 8.17(d), the success rate is high for a narrow groove because the gap can be ignored. Moreover, it is high for a wide groove because the height of the step difference can be ignored. However, for a groove with an intermediate width, it is difficult for the gripper to adhere to the bottom of the groove; hence, the success rate decreases.

When the surfaces of these targets were wetted with water or oil, the gripping success rate increased as compared with those for the dry surfaces. We believe this is because the small gaps between the gripper and the target are filled with fluid.

8.4.3.2 One-acetabulum gripper with a bellows structure

If the target is gripped at a location other than the center of gravity, then the target will easily come off because it will tilt and generate a moment that will separate the target from the gripper. To address this problem, we developed a single gripper with a bellows structure, as shown in Fig. 8.18.

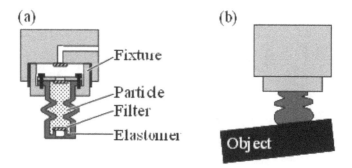

Figure 8.18 A single gripper with a bellows structure.

Figure 8.19 shows the manufacturing procedure for the gripper. The cup-shaped elastomer that has a bellows structure is made of KE-1308 (Shin-Etsu Chemical Co., Ltd.), and we molded it using the metal molds shown in Fig. 8.20. We formed a Teflon film on the mold as a release agent. We mixed the main ingredient KE-1308 with a hardening agent in the standard ratio and poured the mixture into the mold. Then, we filled the cup with glass beads. Finally, we fixed the gripper on a jig. The manufactured gripper is shown in Fig. 8.21.

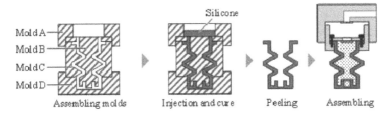

Figure 8.19 Manufacturing procedure for the gripper.

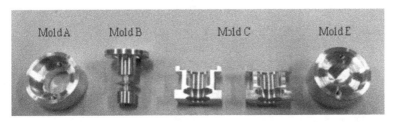

Figure 8.20 Photograph of metal molds into which the silicone rubber is poured.

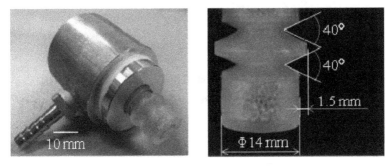

Figure 8.21 The manufactured gripper with a bellows structure.

To determine the relationship between the moment and separation, we investigated the gripping success rate as a function of the gripping location of a flat plate. We pressed the gripper against the target with a constant pressing force (8 N). The target was a flat aluminum plate (100 × 30 × 5 mm, 40 g). We performed the experiment ten times. The conditions for success were that the posture could be maintained for 10 s after suction and lifting.

Figure 8.22 shows the relationship between the gripping location and gripping success rate. For a gripper without a bellows structure, the gripping success rate was 100% when the distance between the center of gravity and gripping location was at most 15 mm. However, for a gripper with a bellows structure, the gripping success rate was 100% for a distance of up to 33 mm between the center of gravity and gripping location. This shows that with a bellows structure, the suction can be maintained even if a moment is generated after suction.

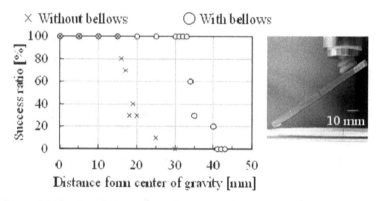

Figure 8.22 The relationship between the gripping location and gripping success rate (left) and the photograph of experiment.

8.5 An Antibacterial Nanosurface Mimicking Cicada's Wing Using Biomimetics

8.5.1 Introduction

The wings of insects such as cicadas and dragonflies have a structure of innumerable pillars with dimensions of the order of nanometers. These unique structures are formed by self-organization. In addition, nanopillar structures are water resistant due to the lotus effect and do not reflect light. Moreover, it has recently been reported that the nanopillar structure shows physical bactericidal action [31]. The currently used antibacterial agents work by chemical action. This is a problem since materials such as Ag ions that show antibacterial action have poor persistent bactericidal ability. However, the antibacterial action of a cicada's wings is persistent due to the nanosurface structure, which has been reported to have a high bactericidal ability of up to kill 450,000 bacteria/(cm$^2 \cdot$min) [32]. In this research, to mimic this nanostructure having such excellent characteristics, we manufactured a low-cost, homogeneous nanosurface structure using a Si substrate [33].

8.5.2 Observational Results of Cicada Wings and Manufacturing of a Sample

We collected cicadas called *kumazemi* (*Cryptotympana facialis*) within the university. We observed the wing surface using a SEM as shown in Fig. 8.23. The average height, width, and pitch of the wings of three cicadas measured randomly were 229, 148, and 196 nm, respectively. Targeting these dimensions, we manufactured Si nanowires using a metal-assisted etching method.

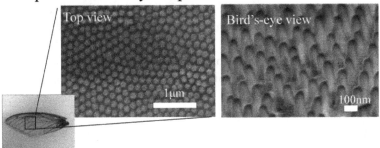

Figure 8.23 The SEM images of a cicada wing surface.

We explain the process, which is shown in Fig. 8.24. We coated and arranged polystyrene spheres with a diameter of 200 nm on a (100) surface of Si substrate using the spin-coating method.

We controlled the particle diameters by ashing with an oxygen plasma. Then, we used the sputtering method to deposit approximately 30 nm of gold. Using gold as a catalyst, we performed Si etching using 15% hydrofluoric acid. Finally, we eliminated the gold and polystyrene spheres to obtain a sample mimicking a cicada wing. The SEM image in Fig. 8.24 shows the manufactured Si nanowires with a height of 200 nm, width of 180 nm, and pitch of 200 nm; hence, we succeeded in mimicking the nanostructure of the cicada wing.

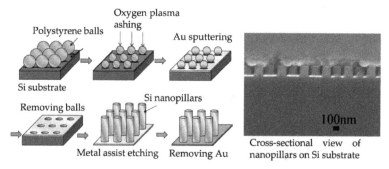

Figure 8.24 Manufacturing process (left) and manufactured wing (right).

8.5.3 Evaluation of Antibacterial Characteristics

In this research, we fixed the pitch as 200 nm and changed the etching conditions to change the height (h) and radius (d) of the nanopillars. In addition, we prepared two types of sample surfaces. One surface had a natural oxide layer (SiO_2), while the natural oxide layer was removed from the other surface (Si).

We evaluated the antibacterial characteristics according to JIS Z 2801. We used a *E. coli* (NBR 3972) bacterial stock suspension, placed a drop (0.3 mL) of the *E. coli* suspension on the manufactured nanosurface sample, covered it with a covering film, and then cultured at 35°C for 24 h. After culturing, we washed the sample surface with 9.7 mL of sterile saline solution, spread the washing liquid on a detection medium sheet for the coliform bacteria group, cultured and counted the number of bacteria, and calculated the concentration of live bacteria after the test.

8.5.4 Results

In the antibacterial characteristic evaluation, we evaluated Si substrates without a nanostructure (with or without a natural oxide layer) as references. Figure 8.25 shows the plot of live bacteria ratio as a function of the height × diameter (= $h \times d$ nm^2) of the nanopillar structure. The live bacteria ratio is the ratio of live bacteria concentration after the completion of the test to the live bacteria concentration immediately after inoculation. A smaller value indicates higher antibacterial characteristics. The detection limit was 10^{-5}.

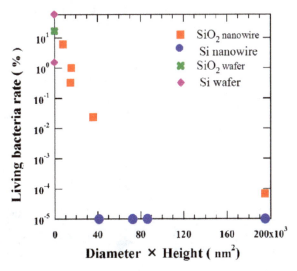

Figure 8.25 The plot of live bacteria ratio as a function of the height × diameter (= $h \times d$ nm^2) of the nanopillar structure.

From the results, we verified that, in the absence of nanostructures on the substrate surface, regardless of the presence of a natural oxide film, the substrate did not exhibit antibacterial characteristics. We also found that the Si surface exhibited excellent antibacterial characteristics independent of the size of the nanopillar structure, while in the case of SiO$_2$ surface, the antibacterial characteristics improved with increasing size in terms of diameter × radius. A Si surface is hydrophobic, while a SiO$_2$ surface is hydrophilic; this suggests that surface hydrophilicity or hydrophobicity has some effects on the antibacterial function.

8.6 Fine Protrusions that Mimic the Footpads of Gecko

8.6.1 Introduction

There is a strong adsorption at the ends of the feet of geckos. This adsorption is due to the van der Waals forces generated by the fine hairs that grow on the footpads of geckos. The van der Waals forces are a type of intermolecular forces, and are strongly exerted when the distance between objects is extremely small [34]. In the foot of a gecko, the van der Waals forces increase because of the fine hairs so that the portion that is in close contact with the target has a larger area. Therefore, we believe that it is possible to manufacture a structure with a high adsorption ability by mimicking the fine hairs on a gecko's feet. The applications of such an adsorption body include a high-function robot hand [35] and adhesive tapes [36].

The fine hairs on a gecko's feet have a two-layer structure. Hairs (spatula) with a diameter of several tens of nanometers branch out on top of one hair (seta) that has a diameter of several micrometers. Figure 8.26 shows the SEM image of an actual gecko hair taken in the laboratory.

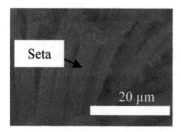
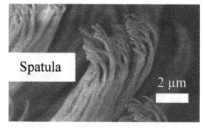

Figure 8.26 The SEM image of an actual gecko hair taken in the laboratory.

8.6.2 Measuring the Adhesive Area of the Footpad of Gecko

We used image analysis to measure the actual area of the adhesive portion of a gecko's foot. Figure 8.27 shows an actual image and the image after binarization. Table 8.1 summarizes the weight of a gecko as measured with an electronic scale (resolution

0.001 g) and the adhesive area of the gecko as determined by the above procedure. We used four geckos for analysis.

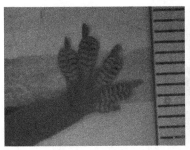 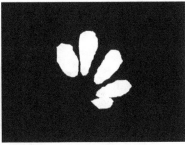

Figure 8.27 Image of gecko's foot. An actual image (**left**) and the image after binarization (**right**).

Table 8.1 The weight of a gecko and the adhesive area of the gecko

Gecko No.	1	2	3	4
Weight gf	3.2	3.9	3.9	4.0
Right fore hand mm²	15.7	19.5	16.0	14.3
Left fore hand	16.4	19.6	15.3	13.6
Right back hand	17.7	22.0	17.5	17.2
Left back hand	20.4	21.9	17.7	17.2
Sum of fore hand	32.1	39.1	31.4	27.9

8.6.3 Adsorption Strength Measurement Experiment

We measured the adsorption strength generated by the foot of a gecko [37]. We used a three-dimensional rapid prototyping device (3D printer) to manufacture a cage on which a weight was placed. The weight of the cage was 3.7 g. We made a gecko, whose tail was fixed, to grip the cage, so that the two front feet could grab the cage. Then, we used a triaxial manipulator to lift the gecko, and we considered the grip successful if the cage could be held for 10 s. This experiment is shown in Fig. 8.28. We performed this operation while changing the weight to determine the limit of the adsorption strength of the gecko. During the experiment, the gecko was anesthetized.

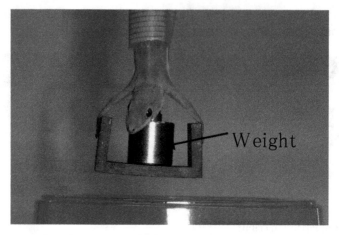

Figure 8.28 Anesthetized gecko holding cage and weight.

The experimental results are shown in Table 8.2. The results for geckos 1 and 2 show that a gecko can lift a weight that is five to seven times its own weight by using just its front feet. In addition, a large difference was observed in the adsorption strength of individual geckos. This may be because the posture made it difficult for the footpads to create adsorption on an object. Another possibility is the dispositions of the gecko's toes. The observations of the usual motions of geckos have shown that the toes are often spread out. However, in this experiment, the toes were contacted with the cage manually; hence, the dispositions of the toes were perhaps inappropriate for exerting sufficient adsorption.

Table 8.2 The limit of the adsorption strength of the gecko

Gecko No.	1	2	3	4
Weight able to lift gf	23.7	18.7	0	3.7

We calculated the adsorption strength per unit area by dividing the adsorption strength exhibited by the gecko in the experiment by the area of the adhesive portion of the footpad as determined by image analysis. As shown in Tables 8.1 and 8.2, although there were individual differences among the geckos, the maximum adsorption strength per unit area was 0.74 gf/mm^2.

For a robot arm, for example the iARM (Exact Dynamics Corp.) that we have in our laboratory, the area of the gripping portion of the robot arm, as evaluated by measuring the dimensions using calipers, is 1.6×10^3 mm². If a gripping structure similar to that of a gecko were provided to this gripping portion, then the generated adsorption strength would be 1.2 kgf. The maximum carrying weight of the iARM is approximately 1.5 kg. Therefore, if the carrying weight is complemented with 1.2 kgf due to adsorption, then its maximum carrying weight can be expected to increase to 1.5 + 1.2 = 2.7 kgf.

8.6.4 Manufacture of an Adsorption Device Using a Three-Dimensional Laser Lithography and Transfer by UV Nano-Imprinting

Using a three-dimensional laser lithography system (Photonic Professional GT, Nanoscribe), we manufactured artificial hairs having a two-layer structure, mimicking the foot of a gecko [38]. We used this as a master, transferred it with a nanoimprinting apparatus (NM-0901HB, Meisho Kiko), and manufactured an adsorption device with a UV-curable resin. In addition, we evaluated the adsorption strength. The detailed methods and results are to be explained in [39].

8.7 A Robot Hand That Mimics the Fingers of a Tree Frog

8.7.1 Introduction

The tree frog lives on trees. It often moves along vertical surfaces or surfaces with large inclines, and to support its body, it creates suction by spreading its fingers, whereas in stable places such as flat areas, it closes its fingers (Fig. 8.29) [40]. In addition, the acetabulum of the tree frog is covered with hexagonal epithelial cells of size 10 to 15 μm surrounded by fine grooves. The surface of each cell is divided into support columns with a diameter of 300 to 400 nm, and is concave [41, 42]. To simplify this mechanism, we substituted a vacuum pad for the biological acetabulum and manufactured a robot hand that could simultaneously create suction and grip, mimicking the motion of the fingers of the tree frog [43].

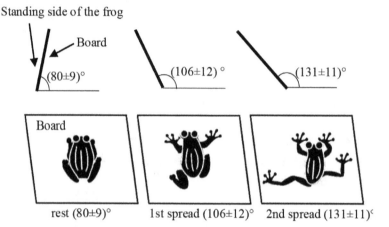

Figure 8.29 The three postures under different degrees of a slanted board [39].

8.7.2 Gripping Strategy

The manufactured robot hand that mimics the hand of the tree frog can grip a target in three ways, which are explained below (Fig. 8.30):

(1) **Gripping a flat target:** The fingers of the robot hand are opened to create suction using the multiple acetabula at the fingertips. By distancing the tips of the three fingers which are the suction points, it is possible to grip stably.

(2) **Gripping a small target:** The fingers of the robot hand are closed to gather the acetabula into one place and grip the target.

(3) **Gripping a target having many curved surfaces:** The target is enclosed with the fingers of the robot hand, and then the interlocking mechanism of the fingers is used to grip along the shape of the target.

A Robot Hand That Mimics the Fingers of a Tree Frog | 179

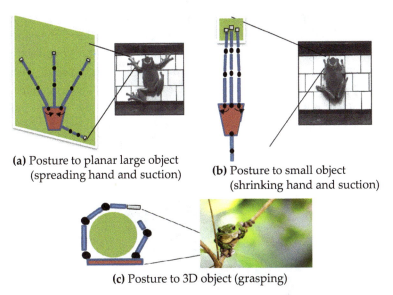

(a) Posture to planar large object (spreading hand and suction)

(b) Posture to small object (shrinking hand and suction)

(c) Posture to 3D object (grasping)

Figure 8.30 The strategy of proposed hand. (left: schematic of hand, right: corresponding frog).

8.7.3 Hand Configuration

Figure 8.31 shows the entire configuration of the robot hand. To simplify the control, the presented robot hand has two degrees of freedom so that it can be driven by two motors. One degree of freedom opens and closes the index finger, middle finger, and ring finger in a flat plane, and the other degree of freedom bends and extends all the four fingers including the thumb. As shown in Fig. 8.32, for the first degree of freedom, we designed an interlocking mechanism that opens the fingers on both sides by using a linear actuator. For the second degree of freedom, we implemented bending and extending operations for all the fingers for adaptive gripping (by bending the joints in sequence starting from the base, the hand moves passively along the target shape) using an actuator (rotary motor), and we designed torsion springs with different spring constants for each joint. A wire goes through each finger, and the motor can wind this to close the hand or loosen it to return the hand to the open condition because of the spring force. The fingertips of the robot hand are provided with multiple suction cup (diameter: 3.5 mm), and suction can be created by using a vacuum generator to generate a negative pressure. The robot hand was manufactured with a three-dimensional printer except for the metal axis portions. The experimentally manufactured robot hand is shown in Fig. 8.33. Figure 8.34 shows the experiments in which three types of targets are gripped by changing the gripping mode.

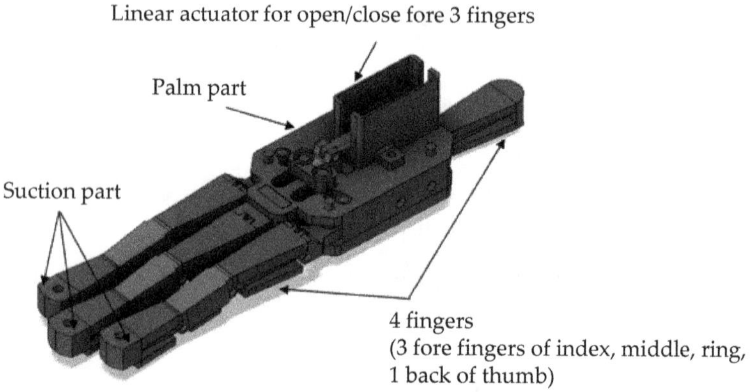

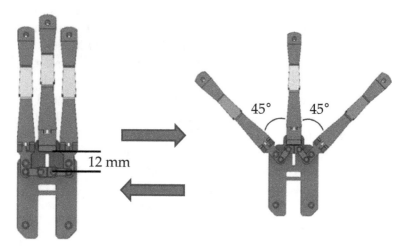

Figure 8.31 The entire configuration of the robot hand.

Figure 8.32 Mechanism to horizontally open fore 3 fingers.

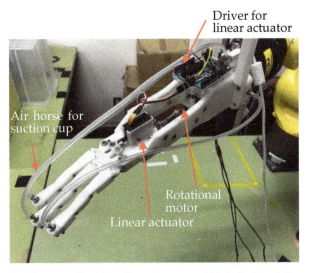

Figure 8.33 Photograph of fore three fingers and their horizontally opening mechanism.

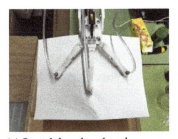
(a) Stretch hand and suck a paper

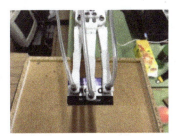
(b) Shrink hand and suck an eraser

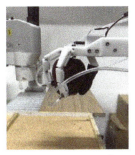
(c) Grasping an apple

Figure 8.34 Experiment of picking object.

8.8 Conclusion

We introduced the biomimetic devices currently under research and development in Kansai University. The shapes of organisms are closely related to their movements, and we believe that in future, the mimicking of not only shapes, but also movements will be important. It is impossible to copy the shapes and movements of animals precisely using the current engineering technology. On the contrary, repeated observations will be necessary to clarify the mechanisms by which functions are expressed, and then come up with ideas to break things down to a level at which the essential features can be extracted and mimicked by technology. To accomplish this goal, cooperation will be needed not only within our specialized field, but also with the people of other fields. This is the difficulty as well as the real charm of biomimetics.

Acknowledgments

This work was supported by the Strategic Research Foundation at Private Universities for the research subject: "Creation of 3D Nano-microstructures and Its Applications to Biomimetics and Medicine" from the Ministry of Education, Culture, Sport, Science and Technology, 2015–2019.

References

1. Shimomura, M. (2010). New trends in new generation biomimetic material technology learned from biodiversity. *Science & Technology Trends*, **110**, 9–28 (in Japanese).

2. Miles, P. (2011). Inspired, naturally, *Financial Times Online*, http://www.ft.com/cms/s/2/37bb18a2-bea7-11e0-ab21-0144feabdc0.html.

3. Aoyagi, S., Izumi, H., and Fukuda, M. (2008). Biodegradable polymer needle with various tip angles and consideration on insertion mechanism of mosquito's proboscis. *Sensors and Actuators*, **A143/1**, 20–28.

4. Izumi, H., Suzuki, M., Aoyagi. S., and Kanzaki, T. (2011). Realistic imitation of mosquito's proboscis: electrochemically etched sharp

and jagged needles and their cooperative inserting motion. *Sensors and Actuators*, **A165-1**, 115–123.

5. Tanaka, T., Takahashi, T., Suzuki, M., and Aoyagi, S. (2013). Development of minimally invasive microneedle made of tungsten—sharpening through electrochemical etching and hole processing for drawing up liquid using excimer laser. *Journal of Robotics and Mechatronics*, **25**, 755–761.

6. Suzuki, M., Sawa, T., Takahashi, T., and Aoyagi, S. (2015). Fabrication of microneedle mimicking mosquito proboscis using nanoscale 3D laser lithography system. *International Journal of Automation Technology*, **9**, 655–661.

7. URL of Robot and Microsystems Laboratory at Kansai University, http://www2.ipcku.kansai-u.ac.jp/~t100051/doc/project_doc3.pdf.

8. Ikeshoji, T. (1993). *Mosquitoes*, University of Tokyo Press, Japan, pp. 189–214 (in Japanese).

9. Oka, K., Aoyagi, S., Arai, Y., Isono, Y., Hashiguchi, G., and Fujita, H. (2002). Fabrication of a micro needle for a trace blood test. *Sensors and Actuators*, **97–98C**, 478–485.

10. Isawa, H., *et al.* (2000). A mosquito salivary protein inhibits activation of the plasma contact system by binding to factor XII and high molecular weight kininogen. *Journal of Biological Chemistry*, **277**, 27651–27658.

11. Nagahama, N., Takahashi, T., Suzuki, M., Aoyagi, S., and Yamamoto, A. (2014). Studies on effect of mosquito saliva on human pain sensation caused by needle puncture (Experiment using an acupuncture needle), in *The 66th Annual Meeting of the Japan Society of Medical Entomology and Zoology*, p. 54 (in Japanese).

12. URL of Terumo Corporation, http://www.terumo.co.jp/.

13. Takayanagi, H., Tanaka, T., Nakao, K., Suzuki, M., Takahashi, T., Aoyagi, S., and Kanzaki, T. (2012). Development of artificial skin using alginate gel and observation of mosquito's penetration. *The 4th Symposium on Micro-Nano Science and Technology*, pp. 259–260 (in Japanese).

14. Wang, J., Oostuki, S., Takahashi, T., Suzuki, M., Aoyagi, S., Kanzaki, T., Kawajiri, Y., and Oono, T. (2014). Fabrication of artificial skin with capillary blood vessels and observation of mosquito bite and sucking blood using it. *Proceedings of the Fall Meeting of Japan Society for Precision Engineering*, 113–114 (in Japanese).

15. Kitada, H., Yamamoto, H., Takahashi, T., Suzuki, M., and Aoyagi, S. (2017). Fabrication of agar inscribed with micro-pitch lattice and observation of mosquito labium motion in puncture. *Proceedings of the Spring Meeting of JapanSociety for Precision Engineering*, 343–344 (in Japanese).

16. Aoyagi, S., *et al.* (2012). Equivalent negative stiffness mechanism using three bundled needles inspired by mosquito for achieving easy insertion, in *2012 IEEE/RSJ International Conference on Intelligent Robots and Systems (IROS2012)*, pp. 2295–2300.

17. Yamamoto, S., Suzuki, M., Takahashi, T., Aoyagi, S., Nagashima, T., Yamaguchi, S., Imazato, S., Kunugi, A., and Saruwatari, T. (2016). Confirmation of cooperative vibration effect of mosquito's mouthpart by non-linear finite element method analysis. *Proceedings of the Spring Meeting of Japan Society for Precision Engineering*, 311–312 (in Japanese).

18. Huang, C., Tanaka, T., Takaoki, Y., Izumi, H., Takahashi, T., Suzuki, M., and Aoyagi, S. (2011). Fabrication of metallic microneedle by electroplating and sharpening of it by electrochemical etching, *IEEJ Transactions on Sensors and Micromachines*, **131**, 373–380 (in Japanese).

19. Gen, H., Sato, J., Suzuki, M., Takahashi, T., Aoyagi, S., Matsumoto, S., Suzuki, K., Ueda, H., Haga, Z., and Miyako, H. (2016). Development of template for microneedle molding using planting technique. *Proceedings of the Spring Meeting of Japan Society for Precision Engineering*, 321–322 (in Japanese).

20. Miyazaki, H., Suzuki, M., Takahashi, T., Aoyagi, S., and Matsumoto, S. (2013). Machining of stainless microneedle with serrations imitating a mosquito and evaluation of its insertion to artificial skin. *Proceedings of the Fall Meeting of Japan Society for Precision Engineering*, 595–596 (in Japanese).

21. Hara, Y., Yamada, M., Tatsukawa, C., Takahashi, T., Suzuki, M., and Aoyagi, S. (2016). Fabrication of stainless microneedle with laser cut sharp tip and its characterization of penetration and blood sampling performance. *International Journal of Automation Technology*, **10**, 950–957.

22. Hara, Y., Yamada, M., Tatsukawa, C., Takahashi, T., Suzuki, M., and Aoyagi, S. (2016). Laser fabrication of jagged shaped stainless microneedle imitating mosquito's maxilla. *International Journal of Automation Technology*, **10**, 958–964.

23. Kier, W. M., and Smith, A. M. (2002). The structure and adhesive mechanism of octopus suckers, *International Society for Computational Biology*, **42**, 1146–1153.

24. Tramacere., F., *et al.* (2013). The morphology and adhesion mechanism of octopus vulgaris suckers. *PLOS ONE*, **8**, 1–7.

25. Horie, T., *et al.* (2007). Micro switchable sucker for fixable and mobile mechanism of medical MEMS, in *Proceedings of IEEE 20th International Conference on Micro Electro Mechanical Systems*, pp. 691–694.

26. Follador., M., *et al.* (2014). Dielectric elastomer actuators for octopus inspired suction cups. *Bioinspiration & biomimetics*, **9**, 046002 (10pp).

27. Hu, B.-S., *et al.* (2009). Bio-inspired miniature suction actuated by shape memory alloy. *International Journal of Advanced Robotic Systems*, **6**, 151–160.

28. Nishita, S., and Onoue, H. (2015). Fluid-filled micro suction-controller array for handling objects, in *The 18th International Conference on Solid-State Sensors, Actuators and Microsystems*, pp. 815–818.

29. Kikuchi, S., Takahashi, T., Suzuki, M., and Aoyagi, S. (2013). Development of flexible vacuum gripper using suction cups for absorbing free-form object, *Proceedings JSME Conference on Robotics and Mechatronics*, 1A1–K03 (in Japanese).

30. Takahashi, T., *et al.* (2015). Vacuum gripper imitated Octopus Sucker-Effect of liquid membrane for absorption, in *Proceedings of IEEE/RSJ International Conference on Intelligent Robotics and Systems*, pp. 2929–2936.

31. Ivanova, E. P., *et al.* (2012). Natural Bactericidal Surfaces: Mechanical Rupture of Pseudomonas aeruginosa Cells by Cicada Wings. *Small*. **8**, 2489–2494.

32. Ivanova, E. P., *et al.* (2013). Bactericidal activity of black silicon. *Nature Communications*, **3838**, 1–7.

33. Ito, T., *et al.* (2016). *Proceedings of IEEE Nano*, 82–84.

34. Autumn, K., Sitti, M., Liang, Y. A., Peattie, A. M., Hansen, W. R., Sponberg, S., Kenny, T. W., Fearing, R., Israelachvili, J. N., and Full R. J. (2002). Evidence for van der Waals adhesion in gecko setae. *Proceedings of the National Academy of Sciences of the United States of America*, **99**, 19.

35. Kim, S., Spenko, M., Trujillo, S., Heyneman, B., Santos, D., and Cutkosky, M. R. (2008). Smooth vertical surface climbing with directional adhesion. *IEEE Transactions on Robotics*, **24**, 65–74.

36. Nitto Denko Corp. (2015). Innovation of adhesive technology by biomimetics-gecko tape using carbon nanotubes. *Journal of the Japan Society for Precision Engineering*, **81**, 385–388 (in Japanese).

37. Sato, J., The, W. W., Takahashi, T., Suzuki, M., and Aoyagi, S. (2017). Production adhesion mechanism imitating gecko by optical shaping and measurement of adhesion force, in *Proceedings of JSME Conference on Robotics and Mechatronics*, 2P1-E11 (in Japanese).

38. Sato, J., The, W. W. Takahashi, T., Suzuki, M., and Aoyagi, S. (2017). Application of gecko adhesive structure to grasping objects, in *Proceedings of JSME Conference on Robotics and Mechatronics*, 2A1-M06. (in Japanese).

39. Terashima, S., Ochi, A., Sato, J., Takahashi, T., Suzuki, M., and Aoyagi, S. Proposal of a three-stage hair structure imitating the sole of gecko foot and its fabrication by UV nanoimprinting. *Precision Engineering*, (in print).

40. Correll, N., Bekris, K. E., Berenson, D., Brock, O., Causo, A., Hauser, K., Okada, K., Rodriguez, A., Romano, J. M., and Wurman, P. R. (2016). Lessons from the amazon picking challenge. *arXiv preprint arXiv*: 1601.05484.

41. Endlein, T., Ji, A., Samuel, D., Yao, N., Wang, Z., Barnes, W. J. P., Federle, W., Kappl, M., and Dai, Z. (2013). Sticking like sticky tape: tree frogs use friction forces to enhance attachment on overhanging surfaces. *Journal of the Royal Society Interface*, **10**.

42. Federle, W., Barnes, W. J. P., Baumgartner, W., Drechsler, P., and Smith, J. M. (2006). Wet but not slippery: boundary friction in tree frog adhesive toe pads. *Journal of the Royal Society Interface*, **3**, 689–697.

43. Jiang, G., Yamagami, S., Takahashi, T., Suzuki, M., and Aoyagi, S. (2018). The proposal of a robot hand for coping with different gripping targets by imitating sucker-attached fingers of tree frogs, in *Proceedings of JSME Conference on Robotics and Mechatronics*, 2P1–F10 (in Japanese).

Chapter 9

Structural Color in Biomimetics

Akira Saito

Department of Precision Engineering,
Osaka University, 2-1 Yamada-Oka,
Suita-si, Osaka 565-0871, Japan
RIKEN SPring-8 Center,
Sayo-gun, Hyogo 679-5148, Japan

saito@prec.eng.osaka-u.ac.jp

The utilization of light by living organisms is superior not only in reaction systems (chemical functions) such as photosynthesis and luminescence, but also in physical functions, and its representative is structural color. Living organisms use structural colors that control color with a micro-/nano-structure in various ways, and it has become clear that light can be effectively utilized with many excellent functions such as non-fading, non-toxicity, material saving, energy saving, and high efficiency. In this chapter, the structural color in biological systems will be summarized, including its applications with concrete examples.

9.1 Introduction

The basis of biomimetics is the excellent characteristics of biological functions, which are summarized in terms of low energy, low environmental load, low cost, and high efficiency.

Biomimetics: Connecting Ecology and Engineering by Informatics
Edited by Akihiro Miyauchi and Masatsugu Shimomura
Copyright © 2023 Jenny Stanford Publishing Pte. Ltd.
ISBN 978-981-4968-10-2 (Hardcover), 978-1-003-27717-0 (eBook)
www.jennystanford.com

Among them, focusing on optical materials, the structural color attracts attention from researchers.

First of all, what is the origin of color? There are multiple principles of occurrence, and the most common source of color is the "pigment." The second most common is "light emission," which is a light source emitting light by itself, such as lighting, fluorescent lamps, lasers and LEDs, etc. In principle, the "pigment" and "emission" are complementary, because the pigment works originally by "absorption" of light (that is, the unabsorbed color appears visible), whereas the light emission is "release" of energy.

However, the third color that is neither "pigment" nor "emission" is a "structural color." As its name suggests, the structural color is a color due to "interference, diffraction, scattering, refraction" of light that is produced by a micro-/nano-structure, and its principle is different from that of "pigment" and "light emission." The optical principles are classified and briefly introduced below.

9.2 Optical Principles

9.2.1 Principles for Structural Color

First, interference (Fig. 9.1(a)) is that the light-waves are intensified (or weakened) according to the optical path, and a specific wavelength (color) is emphasized and a color becomes visible. The optical path is strongly dependent on the structure, which means that "the structure produces color."

Second, diffraction (Fig. 9.1(b)) is originally a phenomenon that a wave hits a structure such as an object or void and goes around it. On the other hand, due to the periodic arrangement of the structures, mutual interaction occurs and a specific wavelength is emphasized (such as diffraction grating in Fig. 9.1(b)). The point that the constructive condition depends on the optical path is common to the interference.

Third, refraction and scattering have more auxiliary roles than interference or diffraction, but they are mentioned as contributions to the structural color. Refraction is well known that the prisms split white light into rainbow colors (Fig. 9.1(c)). Also in this case, there is an effect of changing the color depending on the angle, and the incident and refraction angles depend on the shape of the structure, then it can produce a "structural color."

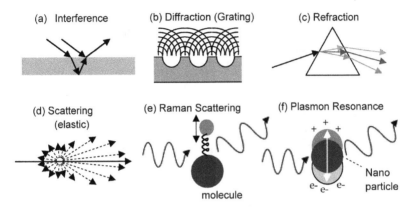

Figure 9.1 Schematic view of principal optical principles to produce the structural color **(a)**–**(d)** and other confusing principles **(e)** **(f)** that are not origin of the structural colors.

In scattering (Fig. 9.1(d)), when the structure scatters light, a color appears because the wavelength depends on the size of the structure and scattering angle (e.g., Rayleigh scattering, Mie scattering, etc.). However, in scattering, some cases may be accompanied by energy transfer (e.g., inelastic scattering represented by Raman scattering (Fig. 9.1(e))), and in that case, even if scattering is a color source, it is hard to say that it is a structural color. Certainly, Raman scattering cannot be said as structural color, because it is caused by molecular vibrations.

Nevertheless, in some cases, the energy transfer of scattering may depend on the micro-/nano-structure (e.g., plasmon by metal nanoparticles, etc.), and the resulting color-change is "coloring by structure." Then, is this called a structural color? But, usually it is not. In this case, the color control by colloidal gold is well known as a typical example, but it is almost an independent field as "plasmon resonance" (Fig. 9.1(f)). If we dare to classify this in the field of coloration, it is "structure-dependent" "absorption" and cannot be called the "third color that has neither absorption nor emission."

To help to understand the relationship among different optical principles and structural color by visualizing the arguments, the overall correlation diagram on the optical principles and structural color is shown in Fig. 9.2. The symbols (a)–(f) in Fig. 9.2 correspond to that in Fig. 9.1.

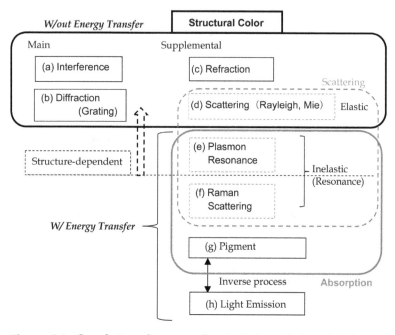

Figure 9.2 Correlation diagram of principal optical principles to produce the structural color **(a)**–**(d)** and other principles **(e)**–**(h)** that are not origin of the structural colors.

Structural colors often have a glittering color with brilliance. This is particularly noticeable in the case of interference and diffraction. The most common examples are soap bubbles and DVD-disk backsides. The former is the result of the interference caused by the thin film thickness, and the latter is of a diffraction grating composed by the tiny hole array. The origin of the glitter is mainly due to the high reflection based on interference and/or diffraction and due to the iridescent effect based on the difference in color angle (also that is called "play color" in the opal that shines with a structural color). However, other factors are also important. Actually, in some cases, the low-reflectance or even a single color can glitter, where several hints of biomimetics are hidden (details will be described from the viewpoint of contrast in Section 9.4).

9.2.2 Types of Structural Color

Figure 9.3 shows the typical principles and structures used for structural color: thin film (Fig. 9.3(a)), multilayer film (Fig. 9.3(b)), opal structure (Fig. 9.3(c)), and liquid crystal (Fig. 9.3(d)). All of them are based on interference and/or diffraction. A typical example of the thin film is the soap bubble, and Fig. 9.3(a) is a schematic view of a commercial pearl material, a representative application of the thin film. It uses the interference in which the surface of micro-flakes of mica is coated with a TiO_2 thin film, and the color can be changed by controlling the TiO_2 film thickness and adjusting the substrate hue [1].

The multilayer film is a common type in structural color such as the bead bug, but in the case of the tropical fish neon tetra, the color can be changed by controlling its angle (Fig. 9.3(b)). The multilayer film on the body of this specie is formed by alternating stack of thin plates of guanine crystals and cytoplasm. Guanine is common in silvery fish and acts as a reflector. Change in color can be realized by controlling the distance (cytoplasmic thickness) and angle of the reflector plate [2].

The opal structure (Fig. 9.3(c)) is one of the most general two structures for the structural color with a multilayer film, and produces color by Bragg reflection based on the crystal arrangement of minute spherical or rod-shaped structures. It is widely found in beetles such as weevil and birds such as peafowl, and the material is silica particles in opal and proteins in organisms [3].

The liquid crystal in Fig. 9.3(d) (cholesteric liquid crystal) forms a helical structure as a result of layered liquid crystal molecules (rod-shaped polymers) being arranged in parallel in each layer and rotating slightly between layers. The incident light causes a kind of Bragg reflection according to the period of the spiral structure, and intensifies the light of a specific wavelength depending on its pitch length and the refractive index. This type of structural color is famous for scarab beetles, and it is known that circularly polarized light is generated depending on the rotation direction of the helix in liquid crystal [4].

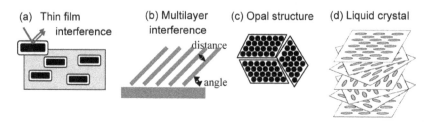

Figure 9.3 Representative structures used for the applications of structural color.

9.3 Applications of Structural Color

9.3.1 Advantages of Structural Color

The structural color is essentially different from the pigment. For example, it can produce a color even when it is made of a transparent material (soap bubbles or DVD is a good example), and the color changes depending on the angle (because optical conditions such as interference change). Furthermore, the structural color is energy-saving compared to light emission, because it does not require self-generated energy. Also it is material-saving, because it does not need a complex synthesis process (the color is determined by physical parameters such as thickness and period, so various colors can be made only by one or two types of materials).

Possibly due to the above-mentioned advantages, structural colors are used in organisms in many cases. It is found from peacocks to tropical birds, many kinds of duck and pigeon, various butterflies, dragonflies, jewel beetles and scarab beetles, tropical fishes typified by neon tetra, and a wide variety of species, with many glittering colors as described above.

The use of structural colors by living organisms is often for the sex selection due to the conspicuous and attracting glitter. However, there are also cases where it is used for mimesis [5] or mimicry [6], which suggests the deep network and functions in natural beings. But, how about the usage by humans?

First of all, there are "brilliant materials" using the glitter, which have wide applications such as cosmetics, decoration, clothing (fiber), etc. In the same direction, the structural color is closely related to the arts, crafts and cultural assets, such as Tamamushi Shrine (7th century) in Horyu-ji Temple, which is miniature shrine that has originally been composed by abundant jewel beetle's wings). Even in posterity, cultural assets and nano-science are deeply related, such as a battle surcoat of samurai warrior that uses many pheasant wings as decoration [7].

Another distinguishing feature of structural color is its anti-fading. In principle, fading is a phenomenon in which a pigment chemically changes by function of UV or oxidation, which leads to discolors. However, the structural color does not fade as long as the physical condition, i.e., the micro-/nano-structure, is maintained. In extreme cases, fossils could keep shining (Scarab beetles of 50 million years ago) [8]. Although the vision system of living organisms varies depending on the species, a theory argues that the original color initially used by living organisms may have been structural color rather than pigment that currently occupies the majority [9]. Certainly, it is possible because the structural color does not require energy transfer nor complex biosynthesis of pigments.

For the important advantage of anti-fade, the application is still interesting. For example, current outdoor posters have faded to gray, and in case of paint, it requires repainting. However, in case of the structural color, the color will be retained even for 1000 years. In addition, there is no environmental load like synthetic dyes, color can be freely controlled by common oxides, and the constituent materials are only 1 or 2 types with different refractive indices. The advantage of controllability only by physical quantities such as thickness and/or refractive index is great.

9.3.2 Various Artificial Approaches

Therefore, the interest in applications of structural color has increased, and many attempts have been made in the last 15 years. The direction of arguments is diverse across principles (Fig. 9.3), materials, manufacture methods, and usages. Since it is impossible to describe everything here, some representative examples will be introduced below. In addition, examples will be given by focusing on biomimetics in consideration with the title and the purpose of the special feature.

The origin of the pearl material in Fig. 9.3(a) is "Raden," which is a technology in ancient times that uses the nacre behind the shells of abalone or pearl oysters. Although the pearl layer of shell is directly inserted in Raden, the pearl material of Fig. 9.3(a) extracted the principle of interference effect and was developed in the United States in the 1960s. It has the advantage of being able to control the color by selecting the base material and changing the film thickness, and is widely used in the paint (mainly automobile) and cosmetic fields.

The multilayer film shown in Fig. 9.3(b) is used in many species such as *Morpho* butterflies and several dragonflies in addition to neon tetra and jewel beetles (pearl also has a multilayer structure), but it is based on a quite common interference effect and in many cases, it is not absolutely derived from organisms (e.g., dielectric mirror, etc.). Meanwhile, a clear pioneer of biomimetics using the multilayer is Teijin's fiber "Morphotex" (released in 2003) [1]. Details will be given in other reports, but there is still a successor in the meaning of multilayer film composed of polymers, "Tetron" from Teijin co. Not only for fibers, it is only necessary to form two layers of materials with different refractive indices into a thin multilayer film, then various applications in both organic and inorganic fields are available.

However, as long as it is an optical thin film, to realize a predetermined hue, it is needed to control the film thickness at the level of several tens of nm, then vacuum evaporation is required and the equipment becomes large, and also high reflectance requires a high refractive-index ratio of two materials (therefore, it is difficult to achieve high reflectance using only resins). Then, there are several restrictions in application of multilayer despite its simple principle.

Recently, a new formation technique of multilayer films, OM (Organized Microfibrillation) has been developed [10]. In OM, a small crack (fibril) layer is formed in a high-density polymer under stress using standing-wave light irradiation and a specific solution preparation. The optical multilayer film is then composed of cracks (air) and polymer layers, and the period can be adjusted by stress, wavelength, solvent, and irradiation time, so that color develops in a wide wavelength range.

In the type of Fig. 9.3(c), colloidal crystals are actively used by artificially accumulating micro-/nano-particles. Various methods have been developed to regularly array the colloidal particles of uniform size [3], whereas as the material, there are choices such as silica and polymer. Because of the difference in reflection depending on the crystal grain boundaries and crystal orientations, color-variations are added to the iridescent color depending on the crystal domain size as well as the colloid particle size.

In consideration of materials, inorganic materials (dielectrics such as metal oxides and silica) or synthetic resins (polyester, polystyrene, PET, etc.) are mainly used either for thin films, multilayer films, or colloids, but for the liquid crystal of Fig. 9.3(d), plant-derived cellulose is also effective. In addition, proteins and chitins are also available for liquid crystal from viewpoint of the rod-shape required for spiral formation (since many basic polymers in living organisms have a rod-like structure, they are compatible with liquid crystal formation). Since the spiral period changes depending on physical conditions (temperature and electric field), wavelength of light can be controlled. Depending on the axial ratio of the unit molecules, there are cases where the liquid crystal formation is triggered by temperature or solution, but both have a disadvantage that it is difficult to fix the color because of the fluidity. However, in a report, helical structure was successfully immobilized using photocrosslinking by synthesis of crosslinkable derivatives [11].

As mentioned above, the discussion of the "structure" and "material" in the structural color is often found in scientific journals, but unexpectedly unknown for the key-point of coloring is the "contrast." To make the structural color (of an organism) look vivid, the point is how to treat the "unreflected colors." If this point is not taken into account, even if a certain color is reflected, its complementary color component is reflected from the background after being transmitted, and the desired color is often whitened. Then what should we do? It is effective to absorb excess color-components using a black background [12], and this technique is frequently found in living organisms.

On the other hand, there is another method to use the molecules and/or the materials itself of the constituent parts being black. In other words, melanin is added to the material, or melanin granules themselves are used as colloids. As a result, a vivid, highly visible structural color is actually produced [13].

Some jewel beetles (multilayer film) and peacocks (micro-particles/rods) actually use melanin pigments effectively, which are examples of deep wisdom of nature.

After discussions on "structure" and "material," "dynamic function" is missing from the above arguments from viewpoint of applications. In addition to decoration and posters, a major potential usage of coloring is dynamic image displays. To change the color dynamically by structural color, the structure or the refractive index should be adjusted by an external stimulus. This requirement is a high barrier on us, but we can find some cues as follows. Biological multilayer films, colloidal crystals, and liquid crystals are often formed by laminating and/or mixing soft tissues based on cytoplasm and solution with hard tissues mainly composed of inorganic substances.

For example, in case of neon tetra's reflector shown in Fig. 9.3(b), their body color is changed by controlling the thickness of the soft tissue composing one part of the multilayer film. Following this, it is possible in principle to control the structure itself, that is, to control the color according to the external stimulus and the environment. Actually, there is an example in which a fine pattern made by semiconductor technology is placed on a gel and color control is shown by changing the salt concentration [14]. However, due to many remaining problems such as change speed and hue control, there is still a distance for practical use.

9.4 "Single Colored" Structural Color: *Morpho* Butterfly

9.4.1 Principles of the Morpho-color

So far, the advantages have been mainly mentioned, but the structural color has a fatal disadvantage: the color changes depending on the viewing angle. In interference and diffraction, wavelengths corresponding to the optical-path difference are intensified. Therefore, if the optical-path difference changes depending on the angle, it is natural that the color changes. Certainly soap bubbles and opals are rainbow-colored and cannot be used for displays such as posters, signboards, and of course, videos.

However, there are species in nature that overcome this difficulty. Some of *Morpho* butterflies, which are representative animals having blue structural color (Fig. 9.4(a)), have an anomalous property of "no viewing-angle dependence" even with interference colors. This is the same as that a soap bubble looks blue everywhere, then this blue is a physical mystery. Therefore, *Morpho* butterflies are not a representative, but exception of the structural color.

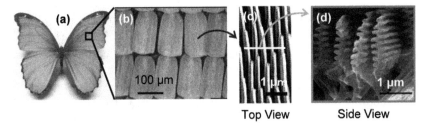

Figure 9.4 (a) Photograph of a representative *Morpho* butterfly (*Morpho didius*), (b) Optical microscopic image of the scales on its wing, (c) SEM image of top view of the scale, (d) SEM image of side view (cross-section) of the scale.

The key to this mystery is the special nanostructure that enables both order and disorder. In brief, the ordered multilayer film gives blue interference, whereas the disorder in structure suppresses interference of other colors [15]. As shown in Fig. 9.4(d), by magnifying their scale (Fig. 9.4(b)), tree-like nanostructures are randomly arranged on the surface of their scale, and each has a narrow multilayer. This tree-shaped multilayer produces a strong blue reflection and the tree-structure's narrow width close to light wavelength produces a wide diffraction spread. As a result of the random arrangement suppressing rainbow interference in oblique light-path, a wide angle and strong blue reflection are realized. Also in the top view as well (Fig. 9.4(c)), a disordered line-shape that is not an ordered line can be recognized, which prevent a grating effect of the ordered line-shape that produces a rainbow coloration.

The principle is surprising, but the greatest attractive point is its potential for application. As mentioned above, the structural color does not fade, is environmentally safe, saves material, and has high brightness. Furthermore, it can be applied to a display because it has single color in wide angular range, and in that case, it is highly energy efficient because of its high reflectance.

Although it is then potentially valuable, there are many obstacles to mass production in controlling the nano-disorder. The authors are progressing with development by overcoming them one by one [16]. The interest in *Morpho*-color is high worldwide, and many attempts to reproduce it have been made.

9.4.2 How to Reproduce the Morpho-color?

The artificial reproduction of *Morpho*-color is based on the fabrication of nanostructures, so it is the question of nanotechnology. In principle, all of three factors, i.e., "1. Periodic structure that causes interference, 2. Narrow tree-width that gives diffraction spread, and 3. Random arrangement that prevents iridescence," are all required. However, realization is often limited to a partial condition (Fig. 9.5(a). The numbers in the figure correspond to that in the above sentence in quotation marks).

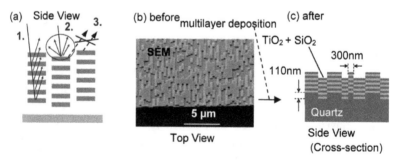

Figure 9.5 (a) Structural model of the *Morpho* butterfly's scale. (1. Multilayer, 2. Diffraction, 3. Disorder to prevent the rainbow iridescence. The numbers correspond to text). (b) SEM image of top view of the artificial *Morpho* plate before multilayer deposition. (c) Schematic view (side view) of the artificial *Morpho* plate after multilayer deposition.

For example, there is a method to use this specie's wing as a template due to the difficulty in producing nanostructures. Atomic layer deposition is used to form an alumina film on the scale and color control is performed by the film thickness [17], or the scale structure were transferred to the polymer (PDMS) by soft lithography [18]. But naturally, there is a problem in productivity because raw wings are required.

Therefore, to complete the process artificially, there are also methods to create a tree structure by lithography and etching: After multi-layered film (SiO_2/Si_3N_4) is lithographically cut into line-shapes, a tree structure was created by selective SiO_2 etching, i.e., multiple-etching [19], or resin molding [20] that evolved from the former technique, also an anisotropic multi-step etching that is composed only of resin [21] were reported. In other example, a three-dimensional periodic structure was obtained by forming an optical interference pattern in a photoresist by interference lithography [22].

The main difficulty for creating *Morpho*-structures is the hierarchical structure consisting of the periodic line structure (trunk of tree-structure in top-view) and fine branches that grow on each trunk (multilayer film in side view). Therefore, in another approach, by using the multi-step nanoimprint lithography (NIL), first, the periodic line of the trunk is formed with shape-memory resin, then it is heated once and flattened, and then a fine structure equivalent to a multilayer film is formed by NIL, and finally the shape is recovered to form a hierarchical structure [23].

However, in all of the artificial processes listed above, the tree structure is created but lacks randomness, and the color's dependence on viewing angle is unfortunately not negligible.

Therefore, in order to introduce randomness, there is an example in which a nano-random substrate is first made of colloidal particles and a blue multilayer film is deposited on it to create a *Morpho*-color [24]. However, the structure was isotropic, and the reflected light was scattered in all directions, which leads to the reflectance per direction decreased.

In two-photon polymerization that can obtain a structure smaller than the light wavelength, a photopolymerization reaction is induced at the laser focus position to draw a three-dimensional structure as designed and a complicated tree structure can be created [25]. However, the drawing speed is slow and productivity is low.

Thus, although many attempts have been made to artificially reproduce *Morpho*-colors, they have not yet been put to practical use. It should be noted that the above examples are limited to the explanation without figures due to the difficulty of copyright permission. If you are interested, please refer to the references.

9.4.3 Another Approach to the *Morpho*-color

Finally, in our method, a quartz substrate was patterned by lithography to mimic the nano-randomness of this specie's scale (Fig. 9.5(b)), on which a multilayer film (SiO_2/TiO_2) was formed (Fig. 9.5(c)). Since the degree of randomness can be "designed," the *Morpho*-color was almost reproduced [16]. By adding laser processing and/or surface-finishing to adjust the disorder, we are progressing toward mass production, but further efficiency could be required depending on the applications.

Efficiency is not the only requirement for realization. "Color design," that is, various simulations for optical effects of nano-randomness [26], and shape control such as powdering and filming are also necessary (but they are also advanced [27]). An additional information on the shape is that the major feature of *Morpho*-color, "single color in wide angle," is much easily realized in the shape of powder than in film. This is because even if the characteristics of one powder particle are "single color in narrow angle," the powder tends to be in a messy direction and thus may give a pseudo-wide angle (Fig. 9.6).

It is easier to make one particle a single color in short wavelength of blue or purple, as compared to red or green. This is because in the case of a multilayer film, the shallower the viewing angle is, the shorter the wavelength appears (when the blue is normal reflection, it looks purple at the shallow angle). In other words, if blue with normal reflection is made with suppression of purple at a shallow angle by adjusting the base material, etc., "at a glance, single blue in wide angle" can be created. There seems to be a similar-type of (self-proclaimed) *Morpho*-color on the market, but "single color in wide angle" of this type is difficult for a single film that is not a collection of powders. Also note that in principle this powder's effect is different from the *Morpho*'s natural skill "to make a wide angle by diffraction spread due to a narrow tree-width" (Fig. 9.5(a)).

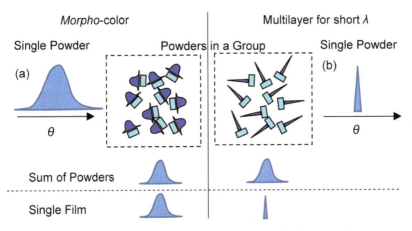

Figure 9.6 Comparison between *Morpho*-color (left) and Multilayer designed for short wavelength (right). (a)(b) comparison of the schematic optical properties (angular reflective profiles) for single powder. (center) image diagram in the form of collective group of powders. (Lower table) comparison of the optical properties under summation of powders (upper) and under a single film.

9.5 New Applications of *Morpho*-Color

The *Morpho*-color was explained so far mainly based on the application of luster materials, but there are new applications that has recently appeared for this decade. It is applications that utilize the nano-hierarchy of their scale structure and is in the field of sensors. Actually, since the reflection spectra change depending on the environment around their scales, it can be used as a sensor by analyzing the reflection (Fig. 9.7).

The pioneering device was gas sensor, which use the change of reflection spectra from the *Morpho* butterfly's scale depending on the atmospheric gas [28]. The spectral modulation is due to the gas-adsorption onto the surface of the tree structure, and if the refractive index varies depending on the gas species, the optical response (reflection spectral modulation) differs, and therefore it becomes detectable. Spectral modulation analysis requires principal component analysis (PCA), a type of multivariate analysis, but it is possible to classify gas species.

Following the elucidation of the analytical principle, an artificial *Morpho*-type gas sensor has recently been demonstrated by functionalizing a tree structure produced by electron beam lithography with polar molecules (trimethoxysilane type) [29]. If gas can be analyzed, a similar analysis can be performed for a higher density phase, i.e., solvent, and some chemical sensors were demonstrated using the fact that the optical response is dependent on the refractive index of filling solvent, such as methanol or ethanol [30].

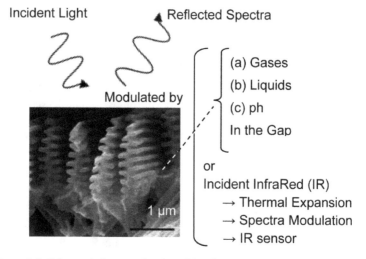

Figure 9.7 Schematic image of various *Morpho*-type sensors.

In addition, as chemical sensors, there are examples of pH sensors [31]. The principle is that the tree structure is surface-modified with "a material that expands and contracts according to pH," then the reflection spectra change depending on the pH value. Since the surface modification is composed of both an acidic layer and a basic layer, the structure of the molecular layer changes depending on the acid or base.

In a sensor application, an infrared (IR) sensor has also been reported [32]. Since the hierarchical tree structure has a large surface area, the addition of carbon nanotubes (CNT) makes it an excellent IR absorber. As a result, IR absorption causes the heated tree structure to expand, changing the reflectance spectrum. An extremely simple and small detector can be configured compared with the conventional IR sensor.

All of these sensors utilize a tree structure, which is the "hierarchical nanostructure" of these species, which suggests that this structure has excellent properties and possibilities. On the other hand, since the structure is hierarchical and then complicated, there is a problem in artificial productivity at present, and future development and industrialization are desired.

9.6 Summary

This chapter argued about the living organism and structural colors, focusing on its relationship with optical materials. However, in the field of structural color, new proposals and discoveries on biological functions are made successively even for the basic principle, not only for the applications. Related researches will be continued actively.

In addition, in the opposite direction from "making color" using the structure, there is another direction, "moth-eye structure" to "erasing color." As the name suggests, the compound eye of the moth has a remarkably low reflectance due to the function of the nanostructure, its application to antireflection coatings is actively developed [1]. Including these broadly defined structural colors, a huge number of hints are probably buried in living organisms, and will be worth watching in the future. Structural color research was pioneered over 300 years ago by pioneers of dynamics, I. Newton [33] and R. Hooke [34]. It continues to provide us with seeds of researches as an endless fountain.

Acknowledgments

This work was partially supported by JSPS KAKENHI Grant Numbers JP26289249, JP19K22062.

References

1. Saito A. (2011). Material design and structural color inspired by biomimetic approach. *Sci. Tech. Adv. Mater.*, **12**, 064709: 1–13.

2. Yoshioka S., Matsuhana B., Tanaka S., Inouye Y., Oshima N., and Kinoshita S. (2011). Mechanism of variable structural colour in the neon tetra: quantitative evaluation of the Venetian blind model. *J. R. Soc. Interface*, **8**, 56–66.

3. Fudouzi H. (2018). Closely packed colloidal crystal assembled with nanoparticles and its application for smart materials with tunable structural color, in *Nanoparticle Technology Handbook* (Naito M., Yokoyama T., Hosokawa K. and Nogi K. eds), Elsevier, pp. 601–605.

4. Mitov M. (2012). Cholesteric liquid crystals with a broad light reflection band. *Adv. Mater.*, **24**, 6260–6276.

5. Saito A. (2019). Biomimetics well understood in biology and engineering 1. *Morpho* butterfly, *Monthly Journal Ohm*, **106** (7), 30–31 (in Japanese).

6. Saito A. (2002). Mimicry in butterflies: microscopic structure. *FORMA*, **17**, 133–139.

7. Museum of Nature and Human Activities, Hyogo (2016)(2019). Temporal Exhibition, "Where culture meets nature" (in Japanese).

8. McNamara M. E., Briggs D. E. G., Orr P. J., Noh H., and Cao H. (2012). The original colours of fossil beetles. *Proc. R. Soc. B*, **279**, 1114–1121.

9. Parker A. (2003). *In The Blink of An Eye*, (Basic Books).

10. Ito M. M., Gibbons A. H., Qin D., Yamamoto D., Jiang H., Yamaguchi D., Tanaka K., and Sivaniah E. (2019). Structural colour using organized microfibrillation in glassy polymer films. *Nature*, **570**, 363–367.

11. Hayata K., Suzuki T., Fukawa M., and Furumi S. (2019). Thermotropic cholesteric liquid crystals from cellulose derivatives with Ester and Carbamate Groups. *J. Photopolym. Sci. Technol.*, **32**, 645–649.

12. Saito A., Murase J., Yonezawa M., Watanabe H., Shibuya T., Sasaki M., Ninomiya T., Noguchi S., Akai-Kasaya M., and Kuwahara Y. (2012). High-throughput reproduction of the *Morpho* butterfly's specific high contrast blue. *Proc. SPIE* **8339**, 83390C: 1–8.

13. Kohri M., Nannichi Y., Taniguchia T., and Kishikawa K. (2015). Biomimetic non-iridescent structural color materials from

polydopamine black particles that mimic melanin granules. *J. Mater. Chem. C,* **3**, 720–724.

14. Shimamoto N., Tanaka Y., Mitomo H., Kawamura R., Ijiro K., Sasaki K., and Osada Y. (2012). Nanopattern fabrication of gold on hydrogels and application to tunable photonic crystal, *Adv. Mater.,* **24**, 5243–5248.

15. Saito A. (2012). *Biomimetic Photonics,* (Karthaus O. ed), CRC Press, Chapter 2. Section 4 "Structural colors" pp. 96–115, Chapter 7. Section 2 "Modeling" pp. 226–242.

16. Saito A. (2019). *Nanoimprint Technology Handbook,* eds. *Jpn. Soc. Appl. Phys.,* Chapter 13, (Ohmsha) pp. 12–16. (in Japanese).

17. Liu F., Shi W. Z., Hu X. H., and Dong B. Q. (2013). Hybrid structures and optical effects in *Morpho* scales with thin and thick coatings using an atomic layer deposition method. *Opt. Commun.,* **291**, 416–423.

18. Kang S. H., Tai T. Y., and Fang T. H. (2010). Replication of butterfly wing microstructures using molding lithography. *Curr. Appl. Phys.,* **10**, 625–630.

19. Aryal M., Ko D. H., Tumbleston J. R., Gadisa A., Samulski E. T., and Lopez R. (2012). Large area nanofabrication of butterfly wing's three dimensional ultrastructures. *J. Vac. Sci. Technol.* B., **30**, 061802:1–7.

20. Tippets C. A., Fu Y., Jackson A. M., Donev E. U., and Lopez R. (2016). Reproduction and optical analysis of *Morpho*-inspired polymeric nanostructures. *J. Opt,* **18**, 065105: 1–11.

21. Zhang S., Chen Y., Lu B., Liu J., Shao J., and Xu C. (2016). Lithographically generated 3D Lamella layers and its structural color. *Nanoscale,* **8**, 9118–9127.

22. Siddique R. H., Hünig R., Faisal A., Lemmer U., and Hölscher H. (2015). Fabrication of hierarchical photonic nanostructures inspired by *Morpho* butterflies utilizing laser interference lithography. *Opt. Mat. Exp.,* **5**, 996–1005.

23. Schneider N., Zeiger C., Kolew A., Schneider M., Leuthold J., Hölscher H., and Worgull M. (2014). Nanothermoforming of hierarchical optical components utilizing shape memory polymers as active molds. *Opt. Mat. Express,* **4**, 1895–1902.

24. Song B., Johansen V. E., Sigmund O., and Shin J. H. (2017). Reproducing the hierarchy of disorder for *Morpho*-inspired, broad-angle color reflection. *Sci. Rep.,* **7**, 46023: 1–8.

25. Zyla G., Kovalev A., Heisterkamp S., Esen C., Gurevich E. L., Gorb S., and Ostendorf A. (2019). Biomimetic structural coloration with tunable degree of angle-independence generated by two-photon polymerization. *Opt. Mat. Express*, **9**, 2630–2639.

26. Saito A., Yonezawa M., Murase J., Juodkazis S., Mizeikis V., Akai-Kasaya M., and Kuwahara Y. (2011). Numerical analysis on the optical role of nano-randomness on the *Morpho* butterfly's scale. *J. Nanosci. Nanotechnol*, **11**, 2785–2792.

27. Saito A., Ishibashi K., Ohga J., Hirai Y., Kuwahara Y. (2018). Fabrication process of large-area *morpho*-color flexible film via flexible nano-imprint mold. *J. Photopolymer Sci. Technol.*, **31**, 113–120.

28. Potyrailo R. A., Ghiradella H., Vertiatchikh A., Dovidenko K., Cournoyer J. R., and Olson E. (2007). *Morpho* butterfly wing scales demonstrate highly selective vapour response. *Nat. Photonics*, **1**, 123–128.

29. Potyrailo R. A., Bonam R. K., Hartley J. G., Starkey T. A., Vukusic P., Vasudev M., Bunning T., Naik R. R., Tang Z., Palacios M. A., Larsen M., Le Tarte L. A., Grande J. C., Zhong S., and Deng T. (2015). Towards outperforming conventional sensor arrays with fabricated individual photonic vapour sensors inspired by *Morpho* butterflies. *Nat. Commun.*, **6**, 7959: 1–12.

30. Yang X., Peng Z., Zuo H., Shi T., and Liao G. (2011). Using hierarchy architecture of *Morpho* butterfly scales for chemical sensing: experiment and modeling. *Sensors and Actuators A*, **167**, 367–373.

31. Yang Q., Zhu S., Peng W., Yin C., Wang W., Gu J., Zhang W., Ma J., Deng T., Feng C., and Zhang D. (2013). Bioinspired fabrication of hierarchically structured, pH-tunable photonic crystals with unique transition. *ACS Nano*, **7**, 4911–4918.

32. Pris A. D., Utturkar Y., Surman C., Morris W. G., Vert A., Zalyubovskiy S., Deng T., Ghiradella H. T., and Potyrailo R. A. (2012). Towards high-speed imaging of infrared photons with bio-inspired nano architectures. *Nat. Photonics*, **6**, 195–200.

33. Newton I. (1704). *Opticks* (Smith & Walford, London).

34. Hooke R. (1665). *Micrographia* (Martyn & Allestry, London).

Chapter 10

Wetting Phenomena on Structured Surfaces: Contact Angle, Pinning, Rolling and Bouncing

Hiroyuki Mayama

Department of Chemistry, Asahikawa Medical University,
2-1-1-1 Midorigaoka-higashi, Asahikawa,
Hokkaido 085-8510, Japan

mayama@asahikawa-med.ac.jp

10.1 Introduction

Various superhydrophobic surfaces can be found in plants and insects [1–15]. In this chapter, we discuss how wetting phenomena correlates with surface structures. Here, we consider two examples. First example is lotus leaf [1–4]. The surface of lotus leaf is fully covered by smaller-sized structures (needle-shaped structures of wax) and larger-sized structures (hemi-sphere structures), where the larger-sized structures are also covered by the smaller-sized structures. Such surface, which has a kind of hierarchical structure, is called "double-roughness structure" (DRS). Water droplets show high contact angle than 150° on lotus leaf with DRS and the water droplets roll down on tilting lotus

---

Biomimetics: Connecting Ecology and Engineering by Informatics
Edited by Akihiro Miyauchi and Masatsugu Shimomura
Copyright © 2023 Jenny Stanford Publishing Pte. Ltd.
ISBN 978-981-4968-10-2 (Hardcover), 978-1-003-27717-0 (eBook)
www.jennystanford.com

leaf with smaller tilting angle smaller than 5°. The rolling water droplets adsorb dusts on lotus leaf and roll out (self-cleaning). Lotus effect thus has both the superhydrophobicity and rolling behavior. Not only this, raindrops are bounced on lotus leaf. On rose petal, similar DRS can be found, however, the smaller-sized structures are wrinkles. On rose petal, water droplets show high contact angle, however, the water droplets strongly stick and do not roll down from rose petal. The reason of the difference in the rolling behavior is resulting from the point whether water droplets penetrate into the spacing between surface structures.

Second example is termite wing [13, 14]. The surface of the termite wing is fully covered by two kinds of structures. One is short needle-shaped structures and other is long needle-shaped structures, where the long needle-shaped structures are not covered by the short needle-shaped structures. It is called "dual surface structure." Such structures are found on the termites which fly in rainy season to avoid predators and to make new nests. It has unique wetting properties that mists are adsorbed, while drizzles and raindrops are repelled. The properties are related to the dual surface structure.

To understand the wetting phenomena on lotus effect and the termite wing, static wetting and dynamic wetting on surface structures should be discussed. The former is directly related to equilibrium contact angle, superhydrophobicity, super-hydrophilicity and pinning effect. The key points are thermo-dynamics based on surface energy and Gibbs free energy ΔG. On the other hand, the latter is the bouncing behaviors of raindrops on the structured surface. The points are Laplace pressure P_L and dynamic pressure P_d for macroscopic droplets, adhesion energy and dissipation energy for smaller-sized droplets from several μm to sub-mm-sized diameter. We describe only the essence of theoretical scenarios here.

10.2 Equilibrium Contact Angle, Wenzel State and Cassie-Baxter State

Usually, the equilibrium contact angle is discussed in terms of the balance of surface tensions between the air-solid interface γ_s, the air-liquid interface γ_L and the solid-liquid interface γ_{SL} at the three phase line of drop on flat surface along the horizontal direction in Fig. 10.1. As a result, the equilibrium contact angle on flat surface θ_f is discussed as Young's relation [16]:

$$\cos\theta_f = \frac{\gamma_S - \gamma_{SL}}{\gamma_L}. \tag{10.1}$$

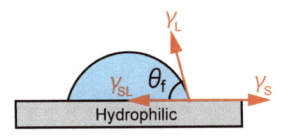

Figure 10.1 Schematic representation of a water droplets on a hydrophilic substrate with flat surface, where the contact angle is θ_f, the air–solid interfacial tension is γ_S, the air–liquid interfacial tension is γ_L, and the solid–liquid interfacial tension is γ_{SL}.

Equation (10.1) is valid for the wetting on flat surface as shown in Fig. 10.2a, but the contact angle depends on surface structure as follows. If liquid fully penetrates into the space between the surface structure as shown in Fig. 10.2b, i.e., Wenzel state, then the contact angle is described by Wenzel's equation [17]:

$$\cos\theta_W = \frac{r_r(\gamma_S - \gamma_{SL})}{\gamma_L} = r_r \cos\theta_f, \tag{10.2}$$

where θ_W is the equilibrium contact angle in the Wenzel state, r_r is the roughness factor and it is the ratio of actual surface area to apparent surface area and $r_r \geq 1$. The contribution of surface structures in wetting is included in r_r. Equation (10.2) means that surface roughness enhances hydrophobicity and hydrophilicity.

If liquid does not penetrate, the wetting state is called "Cassie–Baxter condition" as shown in Fig. 10.2c. Then the contact angle is described Eq. (10.3) [18].

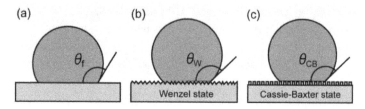

Figure 10.2 Wetting on hydrophobic substrates (a) on flat surface (a), on rough surfaces in Wenzel state (b) and in Cassie–Baxter state (c).

$$\cos\theta_{CB} = f_1 \cos\theta_{1f} + f_2 \cos\theta_{2f}, \tag{10.3}$$

where f_1 and f_2 are the area fractions of the medium 1 and 2 in wetting area and $f_1 + f_2 = 1$, θ_{1f} and θ_{2f} are the equilibrium contact angle of liquid on flat surfaces of the medium 1 and 2, respectively. Assuming that the medium 2 is air (air pocket), then $\theta_{2f} = 180$, $\cos\theta_{2f} = -1$, $f_2 = 1 - f_1$ and $\cos\theta_{CB}$ is

$$\cos\theta_{CB} = f_1 (1 + \cos\theta_{1f}) - 1. \tag{10.4}$$

If the medium 1 is hydrophobic in Eq. (10.4), then $\theta_{1f} < 1$ and the hydrophobicity is enhanced ($\theta_{CB} > \theta_{1f}$).

In the above discussion, the contribution of surface structures in contact angle is included in r_r in Eq. (10.2) and f_1 and f_2 in Eq. (10.3).

10.3 Contact Angle: Thermodynamics of Static Wetting Phenomena

Next, we show that Eq. (10.1) corresponds to thermodynamically stable state in wetting on the basis of interfacial energies and ΔG. Young's relation has been discussed theoretically [19–25], but we simply discussed it based on Gibbs free energy [26]. This is very necessary to consider pinning effect in lotus effect. Actually, Eq. (10.1) is not only the balance condition between γ_S, γ_L, γ_{SL}, but also the thermodynamic stable state as discussed below. Here, it is important to discuss the pinning energy and lotus effect in next section.

ΔG is the difference in Gibbs free energy between before and after wetting and it is formulated as Eq. (10.5).

$$\Delta G = (\gamma_{SL} - \gamma_S)A'_{SL} + \gamma_L(A'_L - A_L), \tag{10.5}$$

where A'_{SL} is the wetting area, A'_L and A_L are the air–liquid interfacial areas after and before wetting. Assuming that the droplets on the substrate are hemispherical geometry as shown as shown in Fig. 10.3. Since the volume of the droplet is constant, then the areas are described by Eqs. (10.6)–(10.8).

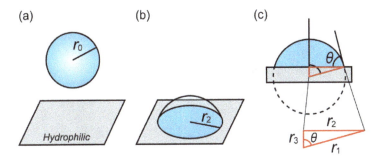

Figure 10.3 Schematic representations of wetting of a water droplet. (a) Before wetting. r_0 is the radius of a spherical water droplet. (b) After wetting. (c) Geometry of the wetting droplet.

$$A'_{SL} = r_r \pi \left(\frac{4}{2 - 3\cos\theta + \cos^3\theta} \right)^{2/3} r_0^2 \sin^2\theta, \tag{10.6}$$

$$A'_L = 2\pi \left(\frac{4}{2 - 3\cos\theta + \cos^3\theta} \right)^{2/3} r_0^2 (1 - \cos\theta), \tag{10.7}$$

$$A_L = 4\pi r_0^2. \tag{10.8}$$

From Eqs. (10.5)–(10.8), ΔG is obtained as Eq. (10.9).

$$\Delta G / 4\pi r_0^2 = [r_r \pi (\gamma_{SL} - \gamma_S)\sin^2\theta - 2\gamma_L(1 - \cos\theta)] \frac{4^{-1/3}}{(2 - 3\cos\theta + \cos^3\theta)^{2/3}} - \gamma_L. \tag{10.9}$$

Equation (10.9) means that ΔG in wetting phenomena depends on θ and r_0 and $\Delta G/4\pi r_0^2$ depends on only θ. The reason why $\Delta G/4\pi r_0^2$ is considered is two-parameter function, $\Delta G/4\pi r_0^2$, is inconvenient to understand the dependence of Gibbs free energy on contact angle, while one-parameter function, $\Delta G/4\pi r_0^2$, is helpful to understand wetting phenomena. The depth of $\Delta G/4\pi r_0^2$ is described by Eq. (10.10).

$$\Delta G/4\pi r_0^2 = 4^{-1/3}(2-3\cos\theta+\cos^3\theta)^{1/3}\gamma_L - \gamma_L. \quad (10.10)$$

Equations (10.9) and (10.10) describe the potential curve and its depth, respectively, as shown in Fig. 10.4. As the condition of free energy minimum of Eq. (10.9), $\partial(\Delta G/4\pi r_0^2)/\partial\theta = 0$, Wenzel's equation is obtained.

$$\cos\theta_{eq} = \frac{r_r(\gamma_S - \gamma_{SL})}{\gamma_L}. \quad (10.11)$$

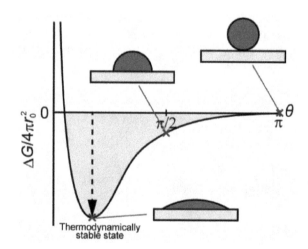

Figure 10.4 Schematic representation of profile of normalized free-energy $\Delta G/4\pi r_0^2$ under a condition of a hydrophilic surface. The shaded area shows wetting state with arbitrary contact angles. The downward arrow shows the thermodynamically stable state, which is described by Young's relation. Even if the contact angle does not reach the equilibrium contact angle, the wetting states in the shaded area are relatively more stable than the state before wetting.

10.4 Pinning Effect

Pinning effect always exist in wetting phenomena on real surfaces. Contact angle discussed in the previous section is one of the important parameters to characterize wetting phenomena, but the pinning effect is also important to understand real wetting such as tear drop-shaped raindrops on window glass. Such wetting is understood by hysteresis of contact angle [12]. This is the difference between advancing and receding angles of droplets on tilting surfaces. In ideal wetting the advancing angle is not equal to the receding angle, however, in real wetting the advancing angle is larger than the receding angle. The hysteresis is observed on both hydrophobic and hydrophilic surfaces, while it is well-known that real surfaces are close to ideal surfaces if the differences are smaller than 5°. In lotus effect, the difference is smaller than 5° on tilting lotus leaf with tilting angle smaller than 5°. Therefore, lotus leaf showing the lotus effect can be considered to be an ideal surface with superhydrophobicity.

The origin of the hysteresis is pinning effect by physical and chemical defects on surface, where the physical defects are surface roughness, while the chemical defects are contamination. Here, let us discuss the pinning effect by physical defects. The point is that the contact line is pinned at the edge of physical defects and the contact angle continuously changes because the edge is included in two surfaces or more. Figure 10.5 illustrates the schematic representation of wetting of a pillar head of a cylindrical pillar. Here, we assume that a water droplet has suitable volume and reaches the equilibrium contact angle θ_f when the water droplet wet the pillar head (Fig. 10.5a,b). Then the contact line of the droplet is pinned at the edge of the pillar. The edge is included in both the pillar head and the pillar side as shown in Fig. 10.5c. The equilibrium contact angle on Surface 1 is θ_f, while the equilibrium contact angle on Surface 2 is $\theta_f + \pi/2$. This means that the equilibrium contact angle continuously changes at the edge between θ_f and $\theta_f + \pi/2$. If the equilibrium contact angle exceeds $\theta_f + \pi/2$, then the contact line moves to the pillar side.

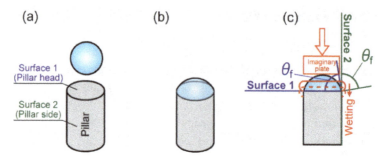

Figure 10.5 Schematic representations of pinning effect. (a) Before wetting of a pillar head of a cylindrical pillar. (b) Wetting of the pillar head. (c) Geometry of a water droplet on the pillar head (side view). Here, it is assumed that the droplet reaches the equilibrium contact angle θ_f when it wets the pillar head.

To evaluate the strength of pinning effect, pinning energy is helpful. This can be evaluated on the basis of ΔG by Eq. (10.5). Ideally, we assume that the droplet on the pillar head is deformed and its shape becomes a pancake and the contact angle of the rim of the pancake for the pillar side reaches $\theta_f + \pi/2$. Since the air-liquid interfacial area is A'_L in Eq. (10.5), it is possible to obtain ΔG and the pinning energy. Skip the detail, but the pinning energy is related to the increase in the surface energy of the pancake-shaped droplet from that of the hemispherical droplet and the pinning energy $E_{\text{full pin}}$ is described by the following equation [26].

$$E_{\text{full pin}} = [(\gamma_{SL} - \gamma_S)A'_{SL} + \gamma_L(A'_L - A_L)]_{\text{pancake}}$$
$$- [(\gamma_{SL} - \gamma_S)A'_{SL} + \gamma_L(A'_L - A_L)]_{\text{hemisphere}}. \quad (10.12)$$

Since the air-liquid interfacial areas before wetting A_L and the wetting areas A'_{SL} are same in Eq. (10.12), Eq. (10.12) is therefore modified as Eq. (10.13) [26].

$$E_{\text{full pin}} = \gamma_L(A'_{L,\text{pancake}} - A'_{L,\text{hemisphere}}), \quad (10.13)$$

where $A'_{L,\text{pancake}}$ and $A'_{L,\text{hemisphere}}$ are the air-liquid interfacial areas of pancake-shaped droplet and hemispherical droplet, respectively. As a result, $E_{\text{full pin}}$ corresponds to the different in the air-liquid interfacial energy in the pancake-shaped droplet and the hemi-spherical droplet.

$E_{\text{full pin}}$ is necessary to discuss the mechanism of rolling or sliding droplet on tilted surfaces in next section.

10.5 Lotus Effect

The surface of raw lotus leaf is fully covered by double-roughness structure consisted of the smaller-sized structures and the larger-sized structures as shown in Fig. 10.6a,b [27]. The smaller-sized structures are made from plant waxes [28]. The waxes are removed by dipping in ethanol for 20 min (Fig. 10.6c,d). On the other hand, the waxes remain during air-drying (Fig. 10.6e,f). The smaller-sized structures made from plant waxes plays a significant role in lotus effect, super water-repellency and rolling behavior of water droplets. For example, it was observed that water droplets on raw and dried lotus leaves (Fig. 10.6a,c) rolls down when lotus leaf is slightly tilted. The angles, rolling angle, are 2.7° and 2.3°, respectively [27]. In contrast, the rolling behavior was not observed on the dipped lotus leaf. The importance of the smaller-sized structures on lotus leaf has been found.

In other experiments, we have observed that water droplets roll down on model surfaces prepared by diarylethene (DAE) derivatives [29–34]. DAEs are known as thermally irreversible photochromic compounds which undergo cyclization reaction by UV irradiation and cycloreversion reactions by visible light irradiation. These reactions occur upon alternate irradiation with UV and visible light [35, 36]. By the cyclization reaction by UV irradiation for suitable period and storage time and temperature after the UV irradiation, needle-shaped crystals and rod-shaped crystals are formed spontaneously. We have succeeded to control the shape of crystals as shown in Fig. 10.7 [29]. The smaller-sized structures play a significant role in rolling behavior, Fig. 10.7b–e shows that the needle-shaped crystals also plays a significant role on single-roughness structure.

216 | *Wetting Phenomena on Structured Surfaces*

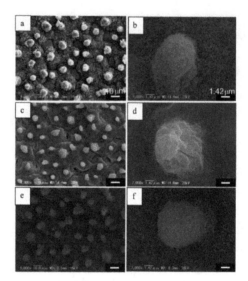

Figure 10.6 SEM images of the surfaces of raw lotus leaf (a, b), lotus leaf after dipping in ethanol for 20 min (c, d) and dried lotus leaf (e, f). Scale bar = 10.0 mm in (a), (c) and (e) and 1.42 mm in (b), (d) and (f). Rolling angles of water droplets on raw and dried lotus leaves are 2.7° and 2.3°, respectively, while water droplets do not roll down on dipped lotus leaf. Reproduced by permission [27].

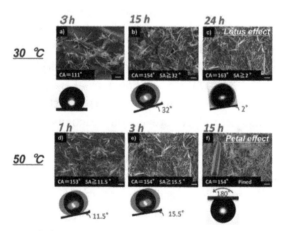

Figure 10.7 SEM images (×2000) of DAE surfaces with different surface structures prepared under different stored temperatures at 30°C (a)–(c) and 50°C (d)–(f) and different stored periods 3, 15 and 24 h (a–c) and 1, 3, 15 h (d–f) after UV irradiation for 10 min. Single-roughness structures (SRS) are observed in (a)–(e). Reproduced by permission [30].

Here, we would like to discuss the mechanism based on a model in which a water droplet exists on slightly tilted multi-pillar surface. Here, essential factors are potential energy ΔU, local pinning energy $E_{local\ pin}$ and adhesion energy E_{ad} [27].

Rolling of droplet seems to be continuous, but we assume that it is discrete as shown as Fig. 10.8. Its driving factor is potential energy ΔU. It is described by Eq. (10.14).

$$\Delta U = mgh \quad (10.14)$$

where m is the mass of the droplet, g is gravitational acceleration and h is the height change by a step h is

$$h = p \sin \phi \quad (10.15)$$

where p is the pitch between ϕ is the rolling angle of slope.

On the other hand, $E_{local\ pin}$ is one of inhibitors and it is the part of $E_{full\ pin}$ as

$$E_{local\ pin} = \frac{d}{2\pi r_2} E_{full\ pin} \quad (10.16)$$

where d is the diameter of a cylindrical pillar. In particular, d is the width of the smaller-sized structure on lotus leaf as shown later.

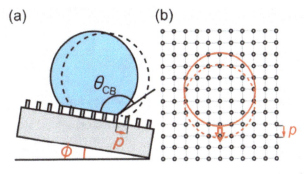

Figure 10.8 Schematic representation of a rolling droplet. (a) Side view. (b) Top view.

In rolling, the dry surface in front of the rolling droplet gets wet, while the wetting surface behind the rolling droplet gets dry. The adhesion energy of the wetting surface by a step is also important as other of inhibitors to understand the rolling behaviors on lotus leaf.

$$E_{ad} = \gamma_L (1 + \cos\theta_r) S \qquad (10.17)$$

where S is the minimum de-adhesion as shown in Fig. 10.9.

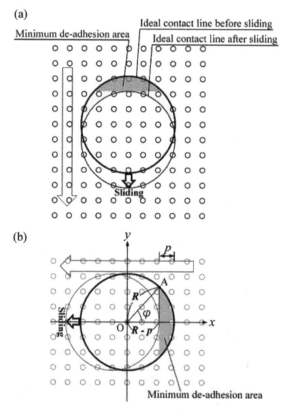

Figure 10.9 (a) Schematic representation of adhesion area along sliding direction and (b) its geometry. Reproduced by permission [27].

$$S = \frac{R^2}{2}(2\varphi - \sin 2\varphi) \qquad (10.18)$$

$$\cos\varphi = \frac{R-p}{R} \qquad (10.19)$$

where R (=r_2) and φ are defined in Fig. 10.9b. Since S depends on the wetting state (the Wenzel state or the Cassie–Baxter state), E_{ad} also depends on the wetting state. In the Cassie–Baxter state, E_{ad} is small.

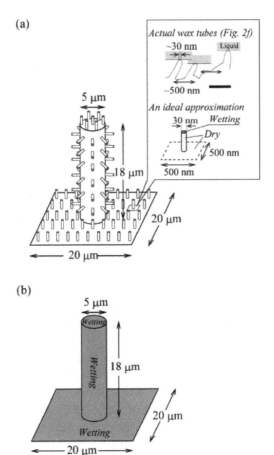

Figure 10.10 (a) Unit of model surface of double-roughness structure of lotus leaf with actual characteristic sizes. The surface is fully covered by the smaller-sized structures and the larger-sized structures. (b) Unit of model surface of lotus leaf after the removal of the smaller-sized structures. Reproduced by permission [27].

Let us discuss the order of ΔU, $E_{local\ pin}$ and E_{ad}. Figure 10.10 shows schematic representation of model surface of lotus leaf with characteristic scales of lotus leaf. In our experiments, the volume of a water droplet was 1.5 μL and $\theta_f = 161°$, $\varphi = 2.7°$, while p between the smaller-sized structure is 20 μm, $d = 30$ nm for raw lotus leaf as shown Fig. 10.10a. Then, it is possible to estimate that $\Delta U \sim$ ca. 7 pJ, $E_{\text{local pin}} \sim 0.75$ pJ, and $E_{\text{ad}} \sim 0.58$ pJ. The smaller-sized structure on lotus leaf has smaller $E_{\text{local pin}}$ and smaller E_{ad} than ΔU, therefore, the water droplets rolled down easily. On the other hand, the water droplets did not roll down on the lotus leaf after the removal of the smaller-sized structures as shown in Fig. 10.9b.

Consequently, it was confirmed that the droplet rolls down if the following conditions are maintained [27].

$$\Delta U > E_{\text{local pin}} + E_{\text{ad}} \tag{10.20}$$

10.6 Bouncing Raindrops on Lotus Leaf: Laplace Pressure and Bouncing Phenomena in Dynamic Wetting of Macroscopic Droplets

Raindrops bounce on lotus leaf. Raindrops bounce on termite wing. This bouncing behavior is important for self-cleaning and non-wetting properties for raindrops. We have succeeded to prepare diarylthene (DAE) surfaces with double-roughness structures mimicking lotus leaf as shown in Fig. 10.11 [32]. We compared the bouncing behaviors of water droplets on lotus leaf, DAE surfaces with single-roughness structure (SRS) and double-roughness structure (DRS) as shown in Fig. 10.11. Water droplets bounced on lotus leaf and the DAE surfaces with DRS (Fig. 10.12a,c), whereas water droplets did not bounce on DAE surfaces with SRS (Fig. 10.12b). To bounce, the air–water interface has to be supported by surface structures and then the Cassie–Baxter state is kept (Fig. 10.12d). To understand the mechanism, Laplace pressure and dynamic pressure are important as discussed below, where the former and the latter are generated by surface structures and the impact of raindrops onto surface. As a result, the raindrops bounce on the surfaces when Laplace pressure is larger than dynamic pressure. Addition to this, the effects of random orientation and length of the smaller-sized structures are discussed.

Bouncing Raindrops on Lotus Leaf | 221

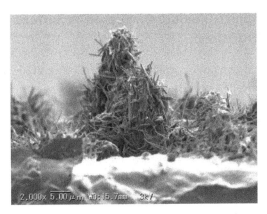

Figure 10.11 SEM images of double-roughness structure of DAE. Reproduced by permission [32].

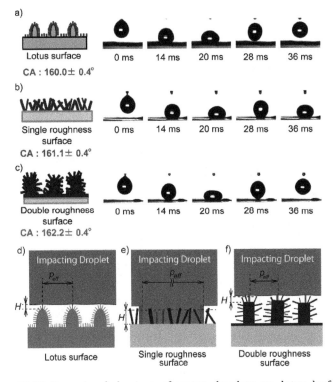

Figure 10.12 Bouncing behaviors of water droplets on lotus leaf (a), single-roughness surface of DAE (b) and double-roughness surface (c). (d) Schematic representations of surface structures and Laplace. Reproduced by permission [32].

10.6.1 Laplace Pressure Generated by Surface Structures

First, let us consider Laplace pressure generated by surface structures. Here, we assume that size of water droplet is macroscopic (mm-scale), while surface structure is μm- and nm-scale and the water droplet exist on multi-pillar surface and its wetting state is Cassie–Baxter state as shown in Fig. 10.13a. The origin of Laplace pressure is the curvature radius R of dipping air–water interface between surface structures in impact (Fig. 10.13b). In principle, Laplace pressure P_L is described by Eq. (10.21) [37]:

$$P_L = \frac{2\gamma_L}{R} \tag{10.21}$$

Considering dipping depth d, dipping angle φ_0 in Fig. 10.13b, we get Eq. (10.22):

$$P_L = \frac{\gamma_L \varphi_0^2}{d} \tag{10.22}$$

Assuming the conditions of $p \gg d$, then P_L is modified as Eq. (10.23) from Eq. (10.22):

$$P_L = \frac{16\gamma_L H}{(\sqrt{2}p - D)^2} \tag{10.23}$$

where H and D are the height and diameter of pillars. Equation (10.23) means that P_L is proportional to H and $(\sqrt{2}p - D)^2$. In other words, P_L reflects the characteristic scales of surface structures. In this discussion, we assume that the standing angle of surface structures (pillars) is always the right angle $(\pi/2)$. Till the situation that φ_0 is larger than the critical angle $\phi_c = \theta_{eq} - \pi/2$ (Fig. 10.13c) the air–water interface is pinned by the edge of pillars. If φ_0 is larger than φ_c, then it advances toward the pillar side.

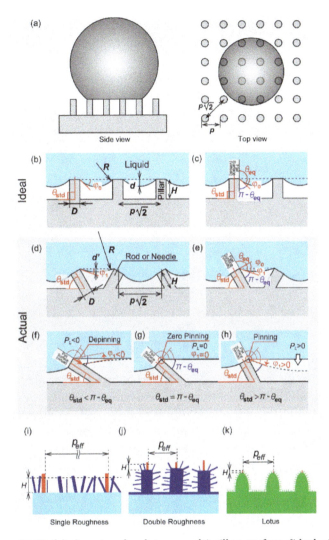

Figure 10.13 (a) A water droplet on multi-pillar surface (ideal single-roughness surface). Left: Side view. Right: Top view of the bottom of water droplet. (b) Schematic representation of dipping air-water interface between pillars. (c) Relationship between equilibrium contact angle θ_{eq}, standing angle θ_{std} and dipping angle φ_0 under the condition that $\theta_{std} = \pi/2$. (d) Relationship between θ_{eq}, θ_{std} and dipping angle φ_1 under the condition that $\theta_{std} < \pi/2$. (f)–(h) Relationship between pinning effect and θ_{std}. (i) and (j) Actual single- and double-roughness surfaces of DAE. (k) Double-roughness surface of lotus leaf. Reproduced by permission [33].

On actual multi-pillar surface, randomly orientated pillars, needle-shaped structures, hairy structures exist. To understand actual Laplace pressure $P_{L,actual}$ generated by such surface structures, it is required to consider how P_L is affected by actual standing angle θ_{std} ($<\pi/2$). Based on Eqs. (10.22) and (10.20), we assume actual standing angle φ_1 and we get $P_{L,actual}$ as Eq. (10.24) [33].

$$P_{L,actual} = \frac{16\gamma_L H}{(\sqrt{2}p - D)^2}\left(\frac{\varphi_1}{\varphi_0}\right)^2,$$

(10.24)

where φ_0 and φ_1 is related to $\theta_{eq}(=\theta_f)$ and θ_{std} as Eqs. (10.25) and (10.26):

$$\varphi_0 = \theta_{eq} - \pi/2,$$

(10.25)

$$\varphi_1 = \theta_{eq} + \theta_{std} - \pi.$$

(10.26)

As a result, it is concluded that $P_{L,actual}$ is proportional to $(\varphi_1/\varphi_0)^2$.

Let us discuss how $P_{L,actual}$ is affected by θ_{std} according to Ref. [33] in which we have succeeded to prepare single roughness surface and double roughness surface using diarylethene derivatives (DAE), a photochromic organic compound. θ_{eq} of DAE is 127°. If θ_{std} is 80°, $P_{L,actual}$ reaches ca. 60% of P_L. If θ_{std} is 70° and 60°, $P_{L,actual}$ reaches ca. 30% and 5% of P_L, respectively. $P_{L,actual}$ thus rapidly decreases when θ_{std} deviates from 90°. These are discussed later.

The above discussion indicates the importance of the standing angle of surface structures on single roughness structure. Contrary to this, the random orientation of surface structure on double roughness structure is acceptable as explained next.

Here, we would like to discuss the relationship between Laplace pressure, SRS surface and DRS surface because this is directly related with H, p and D in Eq. (10.24). SRS surface is the surface covered by a kind of object such as pillars and needle-shaped crystals as shown in Fig. 10.13a,i, therefore, it is simple to relate single-roughness surface, H, p and D in Eq. (10.24).

In contrast, DRS surface is the surface covered by a hierarchical structure as shown in Fig. 10.13k. The DRS surface is covered by smaller- and larger-sized structures and the larger-sized structures are also covered by smaller-sized structures. In this case, it is not simple to relate double-roughness surface, H, p and D because these can be measured from both the smaller- and larger-sized structures and several Laplace pressures can be obtained. However, the advantages of double-roughness surface are that some of the randomly orientated smaller-sized structures on the top of the larger-sized structures stand vertically toward the top and these generate larger Laplace pressure.

10.6.2 Dynamic Pressure

When raindrops collide with lotus leaf, dynamic pressure P_d is generated. It is described by the following equation [37].

$$P_d = \frac{1}{2}\rho V^2 = \rho g h_{\text{release}} \tag{10.27}$$

where ρ is density of liquid (water), V is collision velocity, g is gravitational acceleration, h_{release} is release height of droplet onto surface. This is generated by kinetic energy of falling raindrops.

10.6.3 Bouncing Conditions of Macroscopic Droplets and Importance of Standing Angle and Length of Actual Surface Structures

Let us discuss the relationship between Laplace pressure $P_{\text{L,actual}}$ and dynamic pressure P_d based on the experimental results. In our experiments, water droplets (7.6 µL) were released at different h_{release} (1.8, 50, 100, 150 mm) onto DAE surfaces with single-roughness and double-roughness structures, and lotus leaf. The values of P_d are 17.6, 490, 980, 1470 Pa for h_{release} = 1.8, 50, 100, 150 mm.

On the other hand, let us discuss $P_{\text{L,actual}}$ using Eq. (10.23). $P_{\text{L,actual}}$ of raw lotus leaf (H = 1.7 µm for the smaller-sized structures, D = 0.03 µm for the smaller-sized structures, $p \sim 20$ µm between the larger-sized structures) is estimated to be ca. 2.5 kPa. $P_{\text{L,actual}}$

of DAE with double-roughness structure (H = 3 μm, D = 0.2 μm, p ~ 35 μm) is estimated to be ca. 1.4 kPa. $P_{L,actual}$ of DAE with single-roughness structure (H = 7.6 μm, D = 1 μm, p > 500 μm) is less than 17.6 Pa [32].

In the experiments, water droplets bounced on lotus leaf at $h_{release}$ = 1.8, 50, 100, 150 mm (Fig. 10.12a) and on DAE with double-roughness structure at $h_{release}$ = 1.8, 50, 100 mm (Fig. 10.12c). In contrast, water droplets did not bounce on DAE surface with SRS at all (Fig. 10.12b). These experimental results show that the relationship between $P_{L,actual}$ and dynamic pressure P_d is essential. The bouncing conditions of macroscopic droplets are as follows [32, 37].

$$P_{L,actual} > P_d \tag{10.28}$$

However, fundamental questions, how the standing angle and length of the smaller-sized structures on DRS affect the bouncing behaviors, remained.

In further experiments [33], the fundamental questions were solved as follows. Figure 10.14 shows the relationships between the distribution of the standing angle of the smaller-sized structures and the ratio of actual Laplace pressure to ideal Laplace pressure on SRS surface (Fig. 10.14a), the top of the larger-sized structures (Fig. 10.14b) and the side (Fig. 10.14c) of DAE. Here, θ_{eq} ($=\theta_f$) of DAE was 127° and θ_{rod} ($=\theta_{std}$) 64°. Comparing the distribution shown by the columns and the ratio of Laplace pressures shown by the blue curves by Eq. (10.24), the relationship between the distribution and the bouncing behaviors are unveiled. On DAE surface with SRS, part of the distribution deviates from the blue curve and the part does not generate Laplace pressure as shown in Fig. 10.14a. This explains the reason why water droplets did not bounce on the DAE surface. On the other hand, on the DAE surface with DRS, the distribution matches the blue curve. This explains the bouncing behaviors very much.

Together with the standing angle, the lengths of surface structures are important. The surface structure means the surface structure on the surface with SRS and the smaller-sized structure on the surface with DRS. In the experiments, it is possible to adjust

Bouncing Raindrops on Lotus Leaf | 227

the length of the smaller-sized structure on DAE surface with DRS and we found that the bouncing behaviors strongly depends on the length. If the length was short, water droplets did not bounce. Figure 10.15a shows the experimental results of the bouncing behaviors of water droplets (5.4 µL) at different length of the smaller-sized structure (H_{needle}) and release height ($h_{release}$).

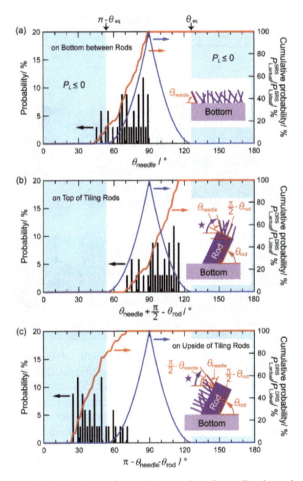

Figure 10.14 Distributions of standing angle of needle-shaped crystals (smaller-sized structures) (columns) and ratio between actual Laplace pressure and ideal Laplace pressure (blue curves) on single-roughness structure (a), top (b) and side of larger-sized structures (c). Here, the observed θ_{rod} (the averages of the standing angle of larger-sized structure) was 64°. Reproduced by permission [33].

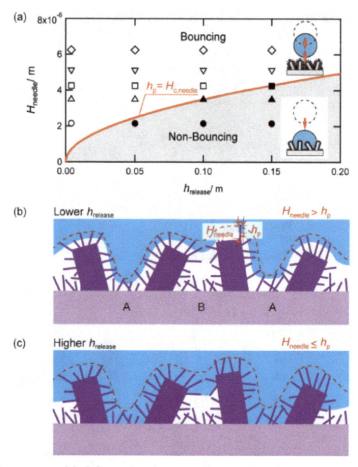

Figure 10.15 (a) Relationship between the length of the smaller-sized structures on double-roughness structures of different DRS (H_{needle}) and the release height ($h_{release}$) of a water droplet (5.4 mL). The open and closed symbols mean bouncing and non-bouncing, respectively. The insets show schematic representations of a bouncing droplet on DRS surfaces with long needle-shaped crystals (upper) and a non-bouncing droplet on DRS surfaces with short needle-shaped crystals (lower). The boundary shown by the red curve is described by Eq. (10.29). (b) and (c) Schematic representations of the relationship between H_{needle} and the penetration depth h_p. The conditions of (b) and (c) are $H_{needle} > h_p$ and $H_{needle} \leq h_p$, respectively. Reproduced by permission [33].

To understand this phase diagram, if we assume that the water droplet behaves as Maxwell model in viscoelastic body at impact, the decay time of tension τ_d depends on viscosity of water η and Young's modulus of droplet. Furthermore, we assume that the air–water interface of the droplet with collision velocity V penetrates into the space between surface structures during τ_d. As a result, it is possible to estimate penetration depth h_p as Eq. (10.29) [33]:

$$h_{\mathrm{p}} = \sqrt{2gh_{\mathrm{release}}}\,\tau_d \qquad (10.29)$$

and

$$\tau_d = \frac{\eta r_0}{6\gamma_{\mathrm{L}}} \qquad (10.30)$$

The red curve in Fig. 10.15a is described by Eq. (10.29). It explains the boundary between bouncing and non-bouncing behaviors very well. If H_{needle} is longer than h_{p}, then the surfaces of water droplets does not reach the bottom between the surface structures and the droplets bounce as show in Fig. 10.15b. In contrast, if H_{needle} is shorter than h_{p}, the surfaces of water droplets reach the bottom and the Wenzel state is realized as show in Fig. 10.15c.

10.6.4 Summary for Bouncing Behaviors of Macroscopic Droplets on Structured Surfaces

In this section, we discussed the bouncing behaviors of macroscopic droplets of water on structured surfaces mimicking lotus leaf. Laplace pressure generated by actual surface structure, dynamic pressure, the standing angle and the length of surface structure play significant roles. Theoretical scenarios explain the experimental results very well. To generate larger Laplace pressure to design bouncing phenomena, smaller p, large H and standing angle close to 90°are essential.

In the above discussion, the bouncing behaviors of macroscopic droplets on structured surfaces are understood on the basis of P_{L} and P_d. Here, it should be noted the size of the macroscopic droplets is several orders of magnitude larger than the spacing between the surface structures and also the dependence of the bouncing behaviors on the size of macroscopic droplets can be neglected because $P_{L,actual}$ and P_d do not depend on the size of droplets. To discuss the size dependence, other theoretical scenario as described below should be considered.

10.7 Bouncing Phenomena of Smaller Droplets on Structured Surface: Restitution Coefficient

As discussed above, the theoretical scenario based on Laplace pressure and dynamic pressure is helpful to understand the bouncing of macroscopic water droplets on lotus leaf. However, it does not work to understand the dependence of bouncing behaviors on the size of droplets such as the bouncing and non-bouncing of μm-sized and sub mm-sized water droplets. The reasons are adhesion energy between droplet and surface structure and dissipation energy induced by deformation of droplets in bouncing. The contributions of these energies are quite different in mesoscopic and microscopic scales. To understand the bouncing behaviors of such smaller-sized water droplets on surface structure is important to understand the wetting phenomena of insects such as termite and mosquitos. For example, termite wing of *Nasuitermes sp.* and *Microcerotermes sp.* adsorb fog (diameter: 1–100 μm), but it repels drizzle (diameter: 100–500 μm) and raindrops (diameter: >500 μm) as shown in Fig. 10.16 [13, 14]. Such wetting property is called "dual wetting." There are two kinds of structures on the surfaces of the wings. As shown in Fig. 10.16a–d, one is a long hair-like projections (macrotrichia) with ca. 50 μm-long and 1 μm-diameter, other is star-shaped projections (micrasters) with ca. 5–6 μm in height and width. Micrasters fully cover the surface at interval of ca. 10 μm, while macrotrichia are sparsely distributed on the surface covered by micrasters at interval of ca. 100 μm.

By photo-induced crystal growth technique for DAE derivatives using UV, we have succeeded to prepare dual surface structure mimicking termite wings as shown in Fig. 10.17 [34]. We adopted two DAE derivatives, DAE 1c and 2c to prepare three kinds of surfaces. The first is **Surf$_{1c}$** by DAE 1c

(Fig. 10.17a,d,g), the second is **Surf$_{2c}$** by DAE 2c (Fig. 10.17b,e,h) and the last is **Surf$_{1c+2c}$** by a mixture of DAE 1c and 2c (Fig. 10.17c,f,i). **Surf$_{1c}$** and **Surf$_{2c}$** are covered by long and short hair-like needles, respectively, while **Surf$_{1c+2c}$** is covered by short and long needles and it looks like the surface structure of termite wings (Fig. 10.16). We estimated that $H \sim 20$ μm for **Surf$_{1c}$**, while $H \sim 5$ μm, $p \sim 3$ μm and $D \sim 3$ for **Surf$_{2}$**.

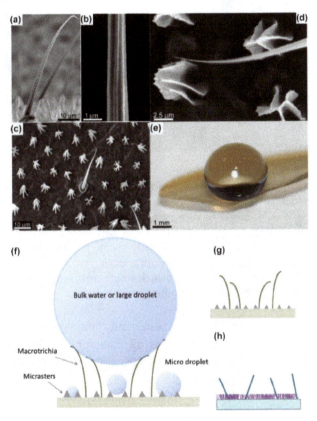

Figure 10.16 SEM and optical images of the termite wing. (a) Side view SEM image revealing hairs (macrotrichia) in sockets protruding from the surface. (b) Expanded SEM image of the macrotrichia revealing a series of nano grooves aligned along the long axis on the hairs. (c) Top view SEM image of the micrasters and macrotrichia on the wing. (d) Expanded SEM image of the termite wing. (e) Optical image of a water droplet on the termite wing. (f) and (g) Schematic illustration of the surface micro-structure of a termite wing. (h) Microcrystalline surface mimicking the termite wing. Reproduced by permission [13].

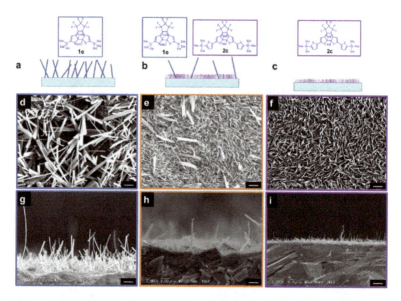

Figure 10.17 Comparison of the photoinduced surface topologies. (a) **Surf₁c**, (b) **Surf₁c+2c**, and (c) **Surf₂c**: pale blue substrate and dark blue crystals correspond to crystals of open- and closed-ring isomers, respectively. SEM images of each surface; (d and g): surface with needle-shaped crystals of **1c**, (e) and (h): surface with needle-shaped crystals of **1c** and **2c**, (f) and (i): surface with needle-shaped crystals of **2c**. Scale bars: 5 mm for (d)–(f) and (h) images, which are magnified 2000 times; 10 mm for (g) and (i) images, which are magnified 1000 times. Reproduced by permission [34]. Comm. Chem.

Using these surfaces, we investigated the bouncing behaviors of smaller-sized droplets in terms of diameter, collision velocity and numbers of bouncing/non-bouncing droplets. Figure 10.18 summarizes the optical images of **Surf₁c**, **Surf₂c** and **Surf₁c+2c**, and also the distributions of the diameter of bouncing/non-bouncing droplets on these surfaces. Obviously, there are two distributions. One is the distribution of non-bouncing droplets in the range of smaller diameter and other is that of bouncing droplets in the range of intermediate and larger diameter. Addition to this, the peak positions are slightly different. Furthermore, the ratio of the number of bouncing/non-bounding droplets is different. The number of bouncing droplets is larger than that of non-bouncing droplets on **Surf₁c**, **Surf₂c** (Fig. 10.18e and f, respectively), whereas the magnitude correlation seems to be reversed on **Surf₁c+2c** (Fig. 10.18g).

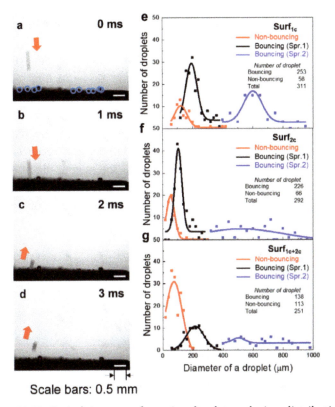

Figure 10.18 Optical images of a microdroplet and size distributions. (a–d) Optical afterimages of the movement of a water droplet during bouncing on **Surf₁c+2c** in 3 ms. Red arrows indicate direction of droplet's movement. Blue circle marks are droplets adsorbing on the surface. (e–g) Distributions of diameters of water droplets contacted with **Surf₁c**, **Surf₂c** and **Surf₁c+2c**. (e) Distribution of diameters of water droplets contacted **Surf₁c**, (f) contacting **Surf₂c**, and (g) contacting **Surf₁c+2c**. In the graphs (e–g), the red dots show diameter distribution of non-bouncing droplets and black dots show diameter distribution of bouncing droplets generated by sprayer 1 (Spr. 1: Generating the microdroplet of 40–400 mm in diameter). The blue dots show diameter distribution of bouncing droplets generated by sprayer 2 (Spr. 2: Generating the microdroplets of 400–1000 mm in diameter). Number of droplets used for preparation of distribution is indicated inside the graphs (e–g). Scale bars for all optical images are 0.5 mm. Reproduced by permission [34].

To understand dual wetting theoretically, it is required to consider the adhesion energy and dissipation energy for macrotrichia and micrasters, where dissipation energy is due to viscous friction in the droplet and it cannot be neglected in bouncing droplets.

To develop this idea, the model as shown in Fig. 10.19 is considered. Before bouncing, we assume that the final velocity of a droplet before bouncing on multi-pillar surface is V, its recoil velocity is V' and the width of a deformed droplet at impact is w, the initial bouncing velocity is v. We skip the detail of the theory, the dissipation energies in impact and recoil and the de-adhesion energy in recoil determines the magnitude of energy loss. To judge whether droplets bounce, restitution coefficient e is useful and it is obtained as the following equation for one surface structure (**Surf$_{1c}$** or **Surf$_{2c}$**).

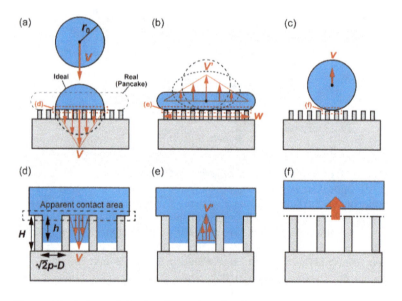

Figure 10.19 A model of a bouncing droplet on multi-pillar surface. Schematic representations of dissipation energy of a droplet before and at impact (a), at beginning of recoil (b) and de-adhesion (c). (d)–(f) Schematic representations of the dissipation energy in the vicinity of the surface structures [34].

$$e^2 = \left(\frac{v}{V}\right)^2 = 1 - \frac{2\eta}{r_0 \rho V}\left[1 + \frac{4r_0^2 V'}{w^2 V}\right] - \frac{3\alpha\pi\eta}{2r_0\rho p^2 V}h^2\left[1 + \frac{V'}{V}\right]$$

$$-\frac{3\alpha\gamma_L(1+\cos\theta_f)}{2r_0\rho V^2}\left(f + \frac{4Dh}{p^2}\right) \tag{10.31}$$

where η is the viscosity of water, ρ is the density of droplets, α is the factor of wetting area for πr_0^2, h is the penetration depth of water between surface structures, f is the area fraction in apparent wetting area in the Cassie–Baxter state, $f = 0.217$ and 0.0816 for **Surf$_{1c}$** and **Surf$_{2c}$**, respectively. D is the diameter of surface structures. The terms including η are related to the dissipation energy. The last term in Eq. (10.31) is due to adhesion energy. V' is determined by Eq. (10.32).

$$(V')^2 = V^2 - \frac{2\eta V}{r_0\rho} - \frac{3\alpha\pi\eta Vh^2}{130} \tag{10.32}$$

On the other hand, the adhesion energy is equal to the energy to peel out a droplet from the surface and it becomes the threshold energy E_{th} to bounce.

$$E_{th} \sim \gamma_L(1+\cos\theta_f)A_{ad} = \alpha\pi\gamma_L r_0^2(1+\cos\theta_f)\left(f + \frac{4Dh}{p^2}\right) \tag{10.33}$$

From E_{th}, the threshold restitution coefficient e_{th} can be obtained.

$$e_{th}^2 = \frac{2E_{th}}{mV^2} \tag{10.34}$$

From Eqs. (10.31) and (10.34), the bouncing conditions are described by Eq. (10.35).

$$e^2 > e_{th}^2 \tag{10.35}$$

236 | *Wetting Phenomena on Structured Surfaces*

The characteristic scales of **Surf$_{1c}$** and **Surf$_{2c}$** are reflected in h, D, f and p in Eqs. (10.31)–(10.33) and the volume of water droplets is included in r_0. This discussion is valid when water droplets bounce on **Surf$_{1c}$** or **Surf$_{2c}$**, not valid on **Surf$_{1c+2c}$**. The reason is that water droplets on **Surf$_{1c}$** or **Surf$_{2c}$** contact with the long needle-shaped crystals of DAE 1c or the needle-shaped crystals of DAE 2c. Contrary to this, water droplets on **Surf$_{1c+2c}$** contact with DAE 1c and 2c at same time or in a very short time.

Considering the restitution coefficient on **Surf$_{1c+2c}$**, the dissipation energy and the adhesion energy are resulting from both **Surf$_{1c}$** and **Surf$_{2c}$**. We get its restitution coefficient of $e_{\text{Surf1c+2c}}$ as Eq. (10.36) although we skip the detail.

$$
\begin{aligned}
e^2_{\text{Surf}_{1c+2c}} = 1 - &\left[\frac{2\eta}{r_0 \rho V}\left(1 + \frac{4r_0^2 V'}{w^2 V}\right) + \frac{3\alpha\pi\eta}{2r_0\rho p^2 V}h^2\left(1 + \frac{V'}{V}\right) \right. \\
&\left. + \frac{3\alpha\gamma_L(1+\cos\theta_f)}{2r_0\rho V^2}\left(f + \frac{4Dh}{p^2}\right) \right]_{\text{Surf}_{1c}} \\
- &\left[\frac{2\eta}{r_0 \rho V}\left(1 + \frac{4r_0^2 V'}{w^2 V}\right) + \frac{3\alpha\pi\eta}{2r_0\rho p^2 V}h^2\left(1 + \frac{V'}{V}\right) \right. \\
&\left. + \frac{3\alpha\gamma_L(1+\cos\theta_f)}{2r_0\rho V^2}\left(f + \frac{4Dh}{p^2}\right) \right]_{\text{Surf}_{2c}}
\end{aligned}
\tag{10.36}
$$

Equation (10.36) means that the dissipation energy is generated by **Surf$_{1c}$** and **Surf$_{2c}$** at same time. The threshold restitution coefficient e_{th}, **Surf$_{1c+2c}$** for **Surf$_{1c+2c}$** is obtained as Eq. (10.37).

$$
e^2_{\text{th,Surf}_{1c+2c}} = \left[\frac{3\alpha\gamma(1+\cos\theta_f)}{2r_0\rho V^2}\left(f + \frac{4Dh}{p^2}\right) \right]_{\text{Surf}_{1c}} + \left[\frac{3\alpha\gamma(1+)}{2r_0\rho V^2}\left(f + \frac{4Dh}{p^2}\right) \right]_{\text{Surf}_{2c}}
\tag{10.37}
$$

As a result, we obtained the conditions of bouncing on **Surf$_{1c+2c}$** from Eqs. (10.36) and (10.37).

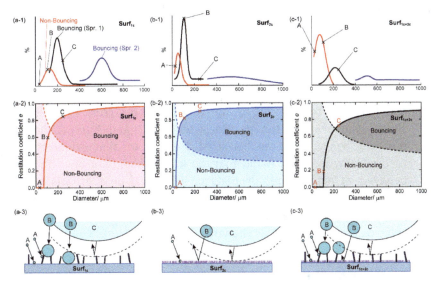

Figure 10.20 (a) On **Surf$_{1c}$**. Schematic representation of distributions of bouncing/non-bouncing droplets on (a-1), calculation results of the bouncing/non-bouncing conditions (a-2) and schematic representation of bouncing/non-bouncing droplets at different diameters (a-3). (b) On **Surf$_{2c}$**. (c) On **Surf$_{1c+2c}$**. In (a-2), (b-2) and (c-2), the calculation conditions are $\eta = 10^{-3}$ Pa·s, $\rho = 10^3$ kg m^{-3}, $V = 1.00$ m s^{-1}, $\alpha = 3.40$, $\theta_f = 130.8°$ and $129.5°$, $f = 0.249$ and 0.0816, $p = 10$ and 3 μm for **Surf$_{1c}$** and **Surf$_{2c}$**, respectively. Point A, B and C in (a-1), (b-1) and (c-1) are plotted in (a-2), (b-2), and (c-2), respectively. Droplet A, B and C in (a-3), (b-3) and (c-3) are corresponding to Point A, B and C, respectively. Reproduced by permission with modifications [34].

$$e^2_{Surf_{1c+2c}} > e^2_{th,Surf_{1c+2c}} \qquad (10.38)$$

To check the validity of theoretical scenario, we compared the calculation results and the experimental results. Figures 10.20a-2, b-2, and c-2 show the calculation results for **Surf$_{1c}$**, **Surf$_{2c}$** and **Surf$_{1c+2c}$**, respectively, where the calculation parameters are shown in the figure caption of Fig. 10.20. In Figs. 10.20a-2 and 10.20b-2, the solid curves are described by Eq. (10.31), while the dashed lines are obtained by Eq. (10.34). These curves are crossing each other and the crossing points rule out the bouncing/non-bouncing behaviors. Non-bouncing occurs in the left areas from the crossing points, while bouncing is observed in the right areas. Similar to this, the solid and dashed curves in Fig. 10.20c-2 are obtained by Eqs. (10.36) and (10.37), respectively. Totally, theoretical diameter ranges of bouncing and non-bouncing droplets are good agreement with the experimental results. Moreover, the experimental results, that the number of non-bouncing droplets on $\mathbf{Surf_{1c+2c}}$ is larger than that on $\mathbf{Surf_{1c}}$ and $\mathbf{Surf_{2c}}$, is reproduced by the result that the cross point is shifted righter than the positions on $\mathbf{Surf_{1c}}$ and $\mathbf{Surf_{2c}}$. The bouncing behaviors of smaller-sized droplets are thus explained theoretically. It is also found that the understanding of bouncing behavior of macroscopic droplets on lotus leaf on the basis of Laplace pressure and dynamic pressure in previous section is valid because the restitution coefficient of mm-sized droplets could be almost constant as shown in Fig. 10.20.

10.8 Conclusion

In this chapter, we roughly discussed from static wetting (the equilibrium contact angle and pinning effect) to dynamic wetting (lotus effect and bouncing droplets) on structured surfaces such as lotus leaf and termite wings. The approaches are based on thermodynamics, Laplace pressure, dynamic pressure, potential energy, kinetic energy, adhesion energy and dissipation energy. Although the detail discussion parts are almost skipped, theoretical approaches, how to solve the fundamental questions how wetting phenomena and surface structure are related, are shown briefly. Here, we focused some wetting phenomena in terms of hydrophobic surfaces. Very recently, we have found that spreading dynamics of water on hydrophilic surfaces is also related to surface structure [38–40]. These are also important to understand wetting phenomena on bio-interfaces such as tongue, fingerprint, small intestine, etc. There are still many questions about the relationship between wetting phenomena and surface structure.

Acknowledgement

I would like to express appreciation to my collaborators, Prof. K. Uchida (Ryukoku Univ.), Dr. R. Nishimura (Rikkyo Univ.), Prof. Y.

Nonomura (Yamagata Univ.), Prof. S. Yokojima (Tokyo Univ. Pharm. Life Sci.) and Prof. S. Nakamura (RIKEN). The studies were supported by JSPS KAKENHI Grand JP18K03554, JP26400424 and JP23540473 in Scientific Research (C).

References

1. Barthlott, W., and Neinhuis, C. (1997). Purity of the scared lotus, or escape from contamination in biological surfaces. *Planta*, **202**, 1–8.

2. Neinhuis, C., and Barthlott, W. (1997). Characterization and distribution of water-repellent, self-cleaning plant surfaces. *Ann. Bot.*, **79**, 667–677.

3. Guo, Z., and Liu, W. (2007). Biomimetics from the superhydrophobic plant leave in nature: binary structure and unitary structure. *Plant Sci.*, **172**, 1103–1112.

4. Wagner, T., Neinhuis, P., and Barthlott, C. (1996). Wettability and contaminability of insect wings as a function of their surface sculptures. *Acta Zool.*, **77**, 213–225.

5. Hensel, R., Neinhuis, C., and Werner, C. (2016). The springtail cuticle as a blueprint for omniphobic surfaces. *Chem. Soc. Rev.*, **45**, 323–341.

6. Otten, A., and Herminghaus, S. (2004). How plants keep dry: a physicist's point of view. *Langmuir*, **20**, 2405–2408.

7. Gao, X. F., and Jiang, L. (2004). Water-repellent legs of water striders. *Nature*, **432**, 36.

8. Lee, H., Lee, B. P., and Messersmith, P. B. (2007). A reversible wet/dry adhesive inspired by mussls and geckos. *Nature*, **448**, 338–341.

9. Feng, L., Zhang, Y., Cao, Y., Ye, X., and Jiang, L. (2011). The effect of surface microstructures and surface compositions on the wettabilities of flower petals. *Soft Matter*, **7**, 2977–2980.

10. Parker, A. R., and Lawrence, C. R. (2001). Water capture by a desert beetle. *Nature*, **414**, 33–34.

11. Bhushan, B. (2016). *Biomimetics*, 2nd ed, Springer, Switzerland, pp. 1–22.

12. de Gennes, P.-G., Brochard-Wyart, F., and Quere, D. (2013). *Capillarity and Wetting Phonomena: Drops, Bubbles, Pearls, Waves*, Springer, New York, pp. 215–259.

13. Watson, G. S., Cribb, B. W., and Watson, J. A. (2011). Contrasting micro/nano architecture on termite wings: two divergent strategies for optimising success of colonisation flights. *Plos One*, **6**, e124368.

14. Watson, G. S., Cribb, B. W., and Watson, J. A. (2010). How micro/nanoarchitecture facilitates anti-wetting: an elegant hierarchical design on the termite wing. *ACS Nano*, **4**, 129–136.

15. Hirose, E., Mayama, H., and Miyauchi, A. (2013). Does the aquatic invertebrate nipple array prevent bubble adhesion? An experiment using nanopillar sheets. *Biology Lett.*, **9**, 20130552.

16. Young, T. (1805). III. An essay on the cohesion of fluids. *Philos. Trans. Soc. London*, **95**, 65.

17. Wenzel, R. N. (1936). Resistance of solid surfaces to wetting by water. *Ind. Eng. Chem.*, **28**, 988–994.

18. Cassie, A. B., and Baxter, S. (1944). Wettability of porous surfaces. *Trans. Faraday Soc.*, **40**, 546–551.

19. Patankar, N. A. (2004). Mimicking the lotus effect: influence of double roughness structures and slender pillars. *Langmuir*, **20**, 8209–8213.

20. Kumar, G., and Prabhu, K. N. (2007). Review of non-reactive and reactive wetting of liquids on surfaces. *Adv. Colloid Interface Sci.*, **133**, 61–89.

21. Marmur, A. (1996). Equilibrium contact angles: theory and measurement. *Colloids Surf. A*, **116**, 55–61.

22. Marmur, A. (1994). Thermodynamic aspects of contact angle hysteresis. *Adv. Colloid Interface Sci.*, **50**, 121–141.

23. Patankar, N. A. (2003). On the modeling of hydrophobic contact angles on rough surfaces. *Langmuir*, **19**, 1249–1253.

24. Nosonovsky, M. (2007). Multiscale roughness and stability of superhydrophobic biomimetic interfaces. *Langmuir*, **23**, 3157–3161.

25. Finn, R. (1986). *Equilibrium Capillary Surfaces (A Series of Comprehensive Studies in Mathematics)*, Springer-Verlag, New York.

26. Mayama, H., and Nonomura, Y. (2011). Theoretical consideration of wetting on a cylindrical pillar defect: pinning energy and penetration phenomena. *Langmuir*, **27**, 3550–3560.

27. Yamamoto, M., Nishikawa, N., Mayama, H., Nonomura, Y., Yokojima, S., Nakamura, S., and Uchida, K. (2015). Theoretical explanation of the lotus effect: superhydrophobic property changes by removal of nanostructures from the surface of a lotus leaf. *Langmuir*, **31**, 7355–7363.

28. Koch, K., Dommisse, A., and Barthlott, W. (2006), Chemistry and crystal growth of plant wax tubules of lotus (*Nelumbo nucifera*)

and Nasturtium (*Tropaeolum majus*) leaves on technical substrates. *Cryst. Growth Design*, **6**, 2571–2778.

29. Uchida K., Nishimura, R., Hatano, E., Mayama, H., Yokojima, S. (2018). Photoresponsive systems mimicking bio-functions. *Chem. A Eur. J.*, **24**, 8491–8506.

30. Nishikawa, N., Mayama, H., Nonomura, Y., Fujinaga, N., Yokojima, S., Nakamura, S., and Uchida, K. (2014). Theoretical explanation of the photoswitchable superhydrophobicity of diarylethene microcrystalline surfaces. *Langmuir*, **30**, 10643–10650.

31. Nishikawa, N., Uyama, A., Kamitanaka, T., Mayama, H., Kojima, Y., Yokojima, S., Nakamura, S., Tsujii, K., and Uchida, K. (2011). Photoinduced reversible topographical change on diarylehthene microcrystalline surfaces with biomimetic wetting properties. *Chem. Asian J.*, **6**, 2400–2406.

32. Nishimura, R., Hyodo, K., Sawaguchi, H., Yamamoto, Y., Nonomura, Y., Mayama, H., Yokojima, S., Nakamura, S., and Uchida, K. (2016). Fractal surfaces of molecular crystals mimicking lotus leaf with phototunable double roughness structures. *J. Am. Chem. Soc.*, **138**, 10299–10303.

33. Nishimura, R., Mayama, H., Nonomura, Y., Yokojima, S., Nakamura, S., and Uchida, K. (2019). Crystal growth technique for formation of double roughness structures mimicking a lotus leaf. *Langmuir*, **35**, 14124–14132.

34. Nishimura, R., Hyodo, K., Mayama, H., Yokojima, S., Nakamura, S., and Uchida, K. (2019). Dual wettability on diaryethene microcrystalline surface mimicking a termite wing. *Comm. Chem.*, **2**, 90.

35. Irie, M. (2000). Diarylethenes for memories and switches. *Chem. Rev.*, **100**, 1685–1716.

36. Irie, M., Fukaminato, T., Matsuda, K., and Kobatake, S. (2014). Photochromism of diarylethene molecules and crystals: memories, switches, and actuators. *Chem. Rev.*, **114**, 12174–12277.

37. Jung, Y., and Bhushan, B. (2008). Dynamic effects of bouncing water droplets on superhydrophobic surfaces. *Langmuir*, **24**, 6262–6269.

38. Nonomura, Y., Morita, Y., Hikima, T., Seino, E., Chida, S., and Mayama, H. (2010). Spreading behavior of water droplets on fractal agar gel surfaces. *Langmuir*, **28**, 16150–16154.

39. Nonomura, Y., Chida, S., Seino, E., and Mayama, H. (2012). Anomalous spreading with Marangoni flow on agar gel surfaces. *Langmuir*, **28**, 3799–3806.

40. Seino, E., Chida, S., Mayama, H., and Nonomura, Y. (2014). Wetting dynamics of colloidal dispersions on agar gel surfaces. *Colloid Surf. B*, **122**, 1–6.

Chapter 11

Powdered Pressure-Sensitive Adhesives Developed Based on Biomimetics

Syuji Fujii[a] and Shin-ichi Akimoto[b]

[a]*Department of Applied Chemistry,*
Faculty of Engineering, Osaka Institute of Technology,
Nanomaterials Microdevices Research Center,
5-16-1 Omiya, Asahi-ku, Osaka 535-8585, Japan
[b]*Department of Ecology and Systematics,*
Graduate School of Agriculture, Hokkaido University,
Kita 9, Nishi 9, Kita-ku, Sapporo, 060-8589, Japan

syuji.fujii@oit.ac.jp

11.1 Introduction

Recent research suggests that organisms first appeared on Earth more than 4.2 billion years ago [1]. It is known from fossils that insects were the first animals that moved from the sea to terrestrial environments, and that they were already present on the supercontinent Pangaea 300 million years ago [2, 3]. Insects and plants underwent explosive radiation and diversified during the Jurassic period and through the Cretaceous period, when the supercontinent separated into continents. The organisms that survived the mass extinction events evolved into what they are today. Incidentally, *Homo sapiens* appeared several hundred thousand years ago.

Biomimetics: Connecting Ecology and Engineering by Informatics
Edited by Akihiro Miyauchi and Masatsugu Shimomura
Copyright © 2023 Jenny Stanford Publishing Pte. Ltd.
ISBN 978-981-4968-10-2 (Hardcover), 978-1-003-27717-0 (eBook)
www.jennystanford.com

Species have evolved and adapted into specific "forms" that are in harmony with their environment by employing complex schemes that have facilitated increased energy savings and efficiency. These evolutionary events have been achieved through trial and error based on the laws of physics and chemistry. The biomimetics refers to the development of products that is based on the morphology/structure, function, and activities of natural organisms. To date, numerous developments have emerged from the biomimetics [4, 5], including hook-and-loop fasteners based on the structure of cockleburs, yogurt lids based on the surface structure of lotus leaves, hypodermic needles based on a mosquito's proboscis, the aerodynamics of the Shinkansen (bullet train) lead car based on the beak of a kingfisher, and swimsuits based on sharkskin.

The authors have developed powdered pressure-sensitive adhesives (PSAs) based on surface and polymer chemistries by mimicking the liquid marble technology employed by aphids [6–8]. The powdered PSAs show no adhesion in its original form and flow like a powder, and show sticky nature only when external mechanical stress is applied. In this chapter, we first explain what liquid marbles are. Then, the fabrication of liquid marbles by aphids in nature, followed by production and characterization of the powdered PSAs, is described.

11.2 What are Liquid Marbles?

Liquid droplets stabilized by solid particles adsorbed at the gas-liquid interface are called liquid marbles (liquid-in-gas type dispersion system), and have diameters in sub-millimeter to centimeter range [9–14]. The driving force for adsorption of particles at the gas-liquid interface is surface free energy. This is because the state in which the particles are adsorbed at the interface is energetically more stable than that in which the particles are not adsorbed at the interface (particles are in gas phase). To fabricate liquid marbles, no electrical power and magnetic field are required; therefore, autonomous energy-saving manufacturing is possible based on the liquid marble technology. Fabrication technology of liquid marbles gives us a chance to re-examine current heteronomous methods of energy-consuming manufacturing under a gravitational force. Thanks to the solid particles adsorbed on the surface of the liquid marbles, the inner liquid does not spread with wetting of the substrate but rolls on it, and the liquid can be taken out by applying external stress.

In recent years, active research with a focus on the properties of liquid marbles has been conducted in the field of physical chemistry. In addition, studies using the liquid marbles as microreactors for cell culture [15], catalytic reactions [16], polymerization reactions [17, 18], and blood-type diagnostic reactions [19], have recently been undertaken. The technology has also been applied to the development of sensors in which either destruction [20–31] or color change [32] occurs in response to external stimulus. Furthermore, a new liquid transport method in which liquid marbles act as carriers was developed [33–39].

11.3 Liquid Marbles Fabricated by Aphids

Liquid marbles may appear to be a new gas-liquid dispersion system; however, if we look to the insect world, we see that aphids have been fabricating liquid marbles [40, 41] since the time before liquid marbles were named by human beings [42].

Aphids, a large insect group, contain about 5000 species in temperate regions around the world [43]. Many of these species are agricultural pests capable of causing extensive damage to crops and trees. Several ant species have been observed to attend aphid colonies. The reason for ant attendance is that aphids excrete sweet wastes called honeydew via their anus as a reward for the protection offered by the ants. Aphids feed on plant sap using straw-shaped mouth parts from highly specialized elongated cells called plant sieve tube elements in the phloem tissue of flowering plants. Phloem sap contains a variety of sugars and amino acids and aphids require these nutrients for their growth and reproduction. Compared with amino acids, the sugar content of phloem sap is high and excess sugar remains even after the nutrients have been metabolized by aphids. Thus, aphids excrete the excess sugar as a viscous droplet of liquid honeydew. Honeydew contains approximately 0.5% to 10%

sugar depending on aphid species. As components of sugars in honeydew, fructose, glucose, and sucrose are the most abundant, and other oligosaccharides, such as melezitose and trehalose are also included [43]. Interestingly, aphids with close symbiotic relationships with ants have been reported to synthesize and secrete melezitose in the honeydew, which the ants prefer [44, 45]. In addition, more than 20 different amino acids have been isolated from honeydew, whose compositions are similar to those of phloem sap [46, 47]. Amino acid profiles in honeydew are reported to change depending on aphid species, seasons or whether the colony is attended by ants or not [48, 49].

Honeydew is excreted from the aphid anus in the form of spherical droplets. If the aphids are tended by ants, these droplets are consumed by the ants shortly after they are excreted. On the other hand, in some aphid species which are not tended by ants, the honeydew droplets are "kicked" far away by the aphids shortly after they have been excreted [50]. This is because honeydew causes a thread against the aphids. If the honeydew, which is a highly nutritious liquid, accumulates on the plant, then it will be utilized by fungi, which could proliferate and block photosynthesis or have some other deleterious effect on the host plant of the aphids.

Aphids of the subfamily Eriosomatinae and Hormaphidinae induce the formation of galls on host leaves in which aphid colonies feed and reproduce [51]. Figure 11.1a shows a gall induced by the aphid *Eriosoma moriokense* on Japanese elm (*Ulmus davidiana* var. *japonica*) leaves. Galls offer the aphids protection and an environment within which to feed on phloem sap. It was reported that the amount of amino acids that had accumulated in the gall was several-hundred fold higher than that in normal leaf tissues [52]. Although the precise nature of this high amino acid concentration mechanism is unknown, inducing galls is a very effective method of concentrating nutrients for feeding. For the aphids that live in galls, the excess amounts of honeydew are problematic. Since ants rarely visit aphids in galls, the honeydew produced by the aphids could either flood the gall or accumulate around the gall, potentially promoting the growth of fungi. In order to solve this honeydew problem, the gall-inducing aphids have developed interesting technology;

they fabricate liquid marbles containing honeydew as the inner liquid.

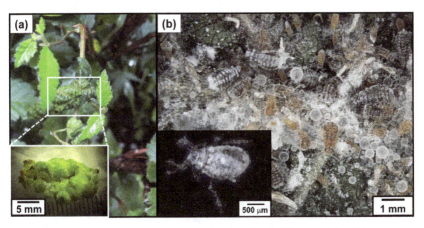

Figure 11.1 (a) Digital camera photograph of gall fabricated by *Eriosoma moriokense* on Japanese elm, *Ulmus davidiana* var. *japonica*. An inset is a magnified image. (b) Stereo microscopy image of inside of the gall. An inset shows an aphid carrying waxes on its back. Reproduced by permission of American Chemical Society.

About 40 species of gall-inducing aphids in Eriosomatinae have been identified in Japan. The bodies of these aphids are covered with white wax fibers that look like cotton (Fig. 11.1b inset). These aphids fabricate liquid marbles by applying the powdery wax to the surfaces of honeydew droplets (Fig. 11.2a,b). As long as the honeydew is kept in this liquid marble state, the honeydew will not stick to the body of the aphid, the gall interior remains clean, and the aphids can move freely inside the gall (Fig. 11.1b). The micrographs in Fig. 11.2a show spherical liquid marbles fabricated by *Eriosoma moriokense* with an average diameter of 368 ± 152 μm (number of measured liquid marbles, 2315) [41] (Fig. 11.2c). The surface tension (γ) and the density (ρ) of the honeydew were determined to be 65.0 ± 4.9 mN/m and 1079 ± 6 kg/m^3, respectively. Using these γ and ρ values, the capillary length (κ^{-1}) was calculated to be 2.48 mm for the honeydew using the following equation:

$$\kappa^{-1} = \sqrt{\frac{\gamma}{\rho g}}$$

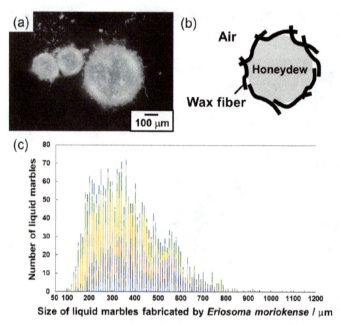

Figure 11.2 (a) Stereo microscopy image and (b) Schematic of liquid marbles fabricated by *Eriosoma moriokense*. (c) Size distribution of the liquid marbles. The number of liquid marbles obtained in the same gall is shown in the same color. Reproduced by permission of American Chemical Society.

The number-average radius of the liquid marbles was one order of magnitude smaller than the capillary length, which indicates that capillaries dominated gravity, and the liquid marble shape is nearly spherical, which accorded well with the results of stereo microscopy observations. The number-average diameter of the aphid anus (D_a) was measured to be 56 ± 13 μm (Fig. 11.3) (number of measured anuses, 188). The honeydew droplet diameter (D_h) was estimated to be 1.27 mm using the following equation by balancing between the capillary and gravitational forces at the aphid anus:

$$D_h = 2^3 \sqrt{\frac{3\gamma D_a}{4\rho g}}$$

The calculated diameter of the droplets was two orders of magnitude larger than the measured diameter. The clear reason is under the veil, but there are two possible reasons: (1) the honeydew droplet expulsion is actively controlled by the opening and closing of the anus, and the drop size could be smaller than that estimated, (2) the shear stress applied to the honeydew droplet attached to the anus during the aphid's movement in the gall.

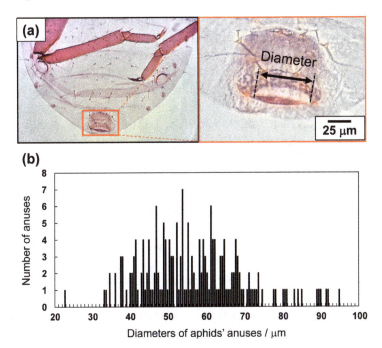

Figure 11.3 (a) Optical microscopy images of anus of *Eriosoma moriokense*. (b) Size distribution of the anuses. Reproduced by permission of American Chemical Society.

Over time, the vibrations of the gall generated by wind, rain and/or animals can cause these liquid marbles to fall through holes in the gall. However, in some aphid species, these holes are very small to prevent attack by predators, and the liquid marbles could not be removed by the vibrations. In such cases, the aphid larvae will actively push the liquid marbles away through the holes with their heads so that the liquid marbles do not accumulate inside the gall [53]. It is interesting to note that the disposal of the honeydew to the outside of the gall is very difficult in a liquid state; however, by fabricating liquid marbles, even small aphids can easily handle a viscous liquid.

11.4 Development of Powdered Pressure-Sensitive Adhesives

PSAs, which are viscous and sticky liquid polymers, are very convenient materials because of their instantaneous bonding characteristics. In daily life, they are used in seals and labels and also as essential materials in advanced industries, including automobiles and electronics. Conventional PSAs are used by applying them to a film substrate (adhesive tape) or by spraying. Although they are useful materials, there are some problems in handling because of their sticky nature, and potential uses are limited. These problems can be resolved if we recall the liquid marbles fabricated by aphids, which are described in the previous section. Aphids prevent the spread of viscous and sticky honeydew inside the gall by fabricating liquid marbles. Inspired by the liquid marble technology of aphids, the authors fabricated PSA liquid marbles with an artificial viscous and sticky polymer core and solid particle shell morphology to produce a powdery PSAs (Fig. 11.4) [6–8]. The specific fabrication method is as follows. First, we fabricated liquid marbles by rolling droplets of an aqueous dispersion of PSA polymer particles on calcium carbonate ($CaCO_3$) powder (primary-particle size: 80 nm) whose surface was hydrophobized with stearic acid. Here, poly(n-butyl acrylate) (PBA), which is popular as one of PSA base polymer, thanks to its optical clarity, stability against UV light and oxidation, and relatively low toxicity and cost, was used as polymer particles. At this stage, a tackifier may be introduced into the liquid marbles as necessary by mixing with the dispersion as an emulsion. The $CaCO_3$ particles immediately coat the droplet of PBA aqueous dispersion and render it both hydrophobic and non-wetting. The resulting liquid marbles remained intact after transferring them onto any substrate including glass and poly(methyl methacrylate). After evaporating water from the latex in the liquid marble, we obtained composite particle (PSA liquid marble), which had the PBA as the core and $CaCO_3$ particles forming the shell. The PBA has a glass transition temperature of –54°C, and it is in a highly viscous and sticky liquid state at room temperature. Because the PBA core is covered with the $CaCO_3$ particle shell, PSA liquid marbles do not stick to substrates. The PSA polymer used as core component is not limited to PBA, and copolymers of n-butyl acrylate and various functional monomers, and other synthetic PSA polymers can also be used. It is possible to drop PSA polymer droplets directly onto the $CaCO_3$ powder to fabricate PSA liquid marbles; however, the viscosity of the PSA is too high and the workability is poor, and it is difficult to fabricate droplets with precise and accurate volumes. Therefore, to fabricate PSA liquid marbles with precise size and size distribution, it is preferable to use an aqueous dispersion of PSA particles with low viscosity. Furthermore, it is possible to control the size of the PSA liquid marble and the weight ratio of the PSA component to the solid particle component simply by controlling the volume of the aqueous dispersion and the solid content concentration. When 15 µL of PBA latex with a solid content concentration of 51% is used, a PSA liquid marble of approximately 3 mm can be fabricated with a weight ratio of PBA and $CaCO_3$ of 94/6. In principle, any solid particles that coat the liquid marble surface can be used as long as their surfaces are hydrophobic. Therefore, the fabrication of PSA liquid marbles is possible utilizing inorganic particles, such as silica and iron and fine organic polymer particles. The assembly of PSA liquid marbles flows down through a funnel and behaves like a flowable powder (Fig. 11.4). When an external stress is applied to the powdered PSA (i.e., the PSA liquid marbles), such as pinching between substrates, kneading with fingers, or screwing, the shell of the PSA liquid marble collapses, exposing the sticky core component inside to the surface, and adhesion is observed (Fig. 11.4).

Compression tests with an indenter confirmed that the PSA core leaks out when the $CaCO_3$ particle shell is ruptured at a compressive stress of 0.14 MPa or more, and the adhesive force increased. The distribution of $CaCO_3$ particles before and after the application of a shear stress to the PSA liquid marble was evaluated with a scanning electron microscopy (Fig. 11.5) and a microfocus X-ray computed tomography system.

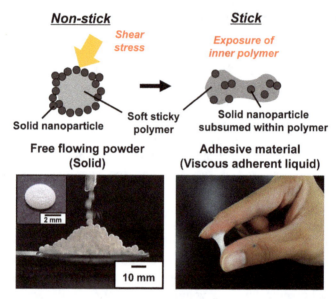

Figure 11.4 Schematic representation of pressure-sensitive adhesion (PSA) powder consisting of particles with soft sticky polymer core and hard nanoparticle shell morphology. After application of shearing stress, adhesion nature appeared because of outflow of inner soft polymer from the hard particles shell. Digital images of such PSA materials are also shown. The PSA shows no adhesion in its original form and flows like a powder. (Inset shows single PSA particle.) Only after application of shear stress it shows its adhesion nature. Reproduced by permission of The Royal Society of Chemistry.

Before kneading, $CaCO_3$ particles are adsorbed on the surface of the PSA liquid marble. On the other hand, after kneading, the $CaCO_3$ particles are partially dispersed in the PSA polymer matrix, and the PSA polymer is exposed to the surface. Tack measurements for one PSA liquid marble were conducted before and after finger kneading (Fig. 11.6). At a pressure of 5.1 kPa, tackiness was hardly detected before kneading (less than 2.0×10^{-3} MPa); however, tackiness appeared after kneading, increasing from 0.05 MPa to 0.35 MPa with an increase of applied pressure. In a control experiment using commercially available PSA tape (Scotch® MagicTM Tape 810), the tack was nearly constant (approximately 0.15 MPa) regardless of applied pressure (Fig. 11.6b). This difference in tack properties between PSA liquid marble and commercial PSA tape is due to the difference in the thickness of the PSA layer. That is, the thickness of the PSA layer is several tens of micrometers in the case of PSA tape, which means that the amount of PSA is too small to wet the whole surface of the substrate with roughness and the contact area on the substrate surface is fixed independent of pressure. In the case of PSA liquid marbles, the adhesive area that wets (contacts) the substrate increases with increasing pressure because the thickness of PSA layer is thick enough (approximately 1 mm). In addition, PSA liquid marbles are very stringy because of the marble thickness, and the peeling energy is higher compared to that of PSA tape.

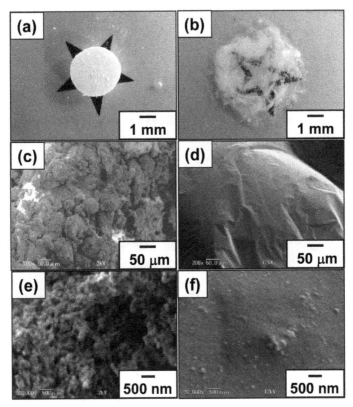

Figure 11.5 (a, b) Digital photographs and (c–f) scanning electron microscopy images of a PSA liquid marble with a soft adhesive PBA core and a CaCO$_3$ hard nanoparticle shell morphology (a, c, e) before and (b, d, f) after application of shear stress. Reproduced by permission of The Royal Society of Chemistry.

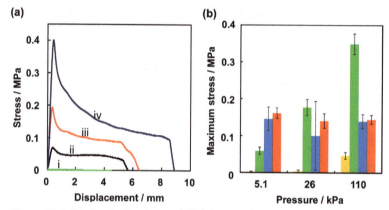

Figure 11.6 (a) Stress-displacement tack curves obtained for PSA liquid marble: (i) before and (ii–iv) after kneading. Pressure applied to PSA liquid marbles: (i, ii) 5.1, (iii) 26 and (iv) 110 kPa. (b) Relationship between pressure applied to PSA materials and maximum stress in tack measurement. Samples: Liquid marble PSA (left bar) before and (left center bar) after kneading, (right center bar) PBA latex film with a thickness of 45 mm and (right bar) commercially available PSA tape (Scotch® Magic™ Tape 810). Reproduced by permission of The Royal Society of Chemistry.

11.5 Conclusions

Liquid marbles fabricated by aphids in the nature, and powdered PSAs developed using the similar principle with the natural liquid marbles based on science and engineering techniques (surface chemistry and polymer chemistry), were described. The fabrication technology of liquid marbles employed by the aphids (at the millimeter-size level where the effect of surface free energy is large) is simple and energy-efficient. In addition, the design method used to fabricate the functional materials is environmentally friendly, as only water, air, and fine particles are used. Adhesion/bonding is a basic industrial technology, and the range of potential applications is very wide. For example, bonding in intricate spaces has become possible using the presently developed powdered PSAs, whereas such applications were not possible using the conventional film or spray-type PSAs. Consequently, the development of new applications of the present PSAs is expected.

Acknowledgments

The authors wish to thank the following individuals: Prof. H.-J. Butt, Dr. M. Kappl (Max-Planck Institute for Polymer Research), Prof. T. Hariyama, Dr. Y. Takaku (Hamamatsu University School of Medicine), Prof. S. Yusa (Hyogo University), Prof. H. Mayama (Asahikawa Medical University), Prof. K. Nakajima (Tokyo Institute of Technology), Dr. S. Deguchi, Dr. S. Okada (Japan Agency for Marine-Earth Science and Technology), Prof. Y. Nakamura, Ms. M. Kasahara, Ms. S. Nakayama, Ms. S. Sawada, Mr. K. Ueno, Mr. K. Shitajima, Ms. N. Karyu, Mr. S. Okada, Prof. T. Hirai (Osaka Institute of Technology) and Sumitomo Chemical for their assistances in characterization of liquid marbles in nature and powdered PSAs. Shiraishi Kogyo Kaisha; Ltd. is thanked for kind donation of $CaCO_3$ nanoparticles. This work was partially supported by JSPS-DAAD Bilateral Joint Research Projects and by a Grant-in-Aid for Scientific Research on Innovative Areas "Engineering Neo-Biomimetics," "New Polymeric Materials Based on Element-Blocks" and "Molecular Soft Interface Science" from the Ministry of Education, Culture, Sports, Science, and Technology of Japan.

References

1. Dodd, M. S., Papineau, D., Grenne, T., Slack, J. F., Rittner, M., Pirajno, F., O'Neil, J., and Little, C. T. S. (2017). Evidence for early life in Earth's oldest hydrothermal vent precipitates. *Nature*, **543**, 60–64.

2. Mori, N., Yoshinaga, N., and Aboshi, T. (2009). Section II Chapter 1 "Konchu-shokubutukan no koubou to syokubutumeneki sisutemu no kaimen," in *Konchu ga Hiraku Miraikagaku* (Fujisaki, K., Nishida, R., and Sakuma, M., eds), Kyoto University Press, pp. 165–189. (in Japanese).

3. Engel, M. S., and Grimaldi, D. A. (2004). New light shed on the oldest insect, *Nature*, **427**, 627–630.

4. Benyus, J. M. (2009). *Biomimicry: Innovation Inspired by Nature*, Harper Collins.

5. Hozumi, A., Jiang, L., Lee, H., and Shimomura, M. (2018). *Stimuli-Responsive Dewetting/Wetting Smart Surfaces and Interfaces*, Springer International Publishing.

6. Fujii, S., Sawada, S., Nakayama, S., Kappl, M., Ueno, K., Shitajima, K., Butt, H.-J., and Nakamura, Y. (2016). Pressure-sensitive adhesive powder. *Mater. Horiz.*, **3**, 47–52.

7. Aron, J. (2015). Powdered glue goes on dry and sticks when squished. *New Scientist*, 16.

8. Fujii, S. (2016). Designing an easy-to-handle powder PSA based on the habits of aphids. *Convertech & e-Print*, **6(4)**, 16–17.

9. Aussillous, P., and Quéré, D. (2006). Properties of liquid marbles. *Proc. R. Soc. A*, **462**(2067), 973–999.

10. McHale, G., and Newton, M. I. (2015). Liquid marbles: topical context within soft matter and recent progress. *Soft Matter*, **11**(13), 2530–2546.

11. Ooi, C. H., and Nguyen, N.-T. (2015). Manipulation of liquid marbles. *Microfluid. Nanofluid.*, **19**(3), 483–495.

12. Fujii, S., Yusa, S., and Nakamura, Y. (2016). Stimuli-responsive liquid marbles: controlling structure, shape, stability and motion. *Adv. Funct. Mater.*, **26**(40), 7206–7223.

13. Bormashenko, E. (2017). Liquid marbles, elastic nonstick droplets: from minireactors to self-propulsion. *Langmuir*, **33**(3), 663–669.

14. Fujii, S. (2019). Stimulus-responsive soft dispersed systems developed based on functional polymer particles: bubbles and liquid marbles. *Polym. J.*, **51**, 1081–1101.

15. Arbatan, T., Al-Abboodi, A., Sarvi, F., Chan, P. P. Y., and Shen, W. (2012). Tumor inside a pearl drop. *Adv. Healthc. Mater.*, **1**(4), 467–469.

16. Wang, D., Zhu, L., Chen, J.-F., and Dai, L. (2016). Liquid marbles based on magnetic upconversion nanoparticles as magnetically and optically responsive miniature reactors for photocatalysis and photodynamic therapy. *Angew. Chem. Int. Ed.*, **55**(36), 10795–10799.

17. Sato, E., Yuri, M., Fujii, S., Nishiyama, T., Nakamura, Y., and Horibe, H. (2015). Liquid marbles as a micro-reactor for efficient radical alternating copolymerization of diene monomer and oxygen. *Chem. Commun.*, **51**(97), 17241–17244.

18. Sato, E., Yuri, M., Fujii, S., Nishiyama, T., Nakamura, Y., and Horibe, H. (2016). Liquid marble containing degradable polyperoxides for adhesion force-changeable pressure-sensitive adhesives. *RSC Adv.*, **6**, 56475–56481.

19. Arbatan, T., Li, L., Tian, J., and Shen, W. (2012). Microreactors: liquid marbles as micro-bioreactors for rapid blood typing. *Adv. Healthc. Mater.*, **1**(1), 80–83.

20. Dupin, D., Armes, S. P., and Fujii S. (2009). Stimulus-responsive liquid marble, *J. Am. Chem. Soc.*, **131**(15), 5386–5387.

21. Fujii, S., Kameyama, S., Dupin, D., Armes, S. P., Suzaki, M., and Nakamura, Y. (2010). pH-responsive liquid marbles stabilized with poly(2-vinylpyridine) particles. *Soft Matter*, **6**(3), 635–640.

22. Inoue, M., Fujii, S., Nakamura, Y., Iwasaki, Y., and Yusa, S. (2011). pH-responsive disruption of "liquid marbles" prepared from water and poly(6-(acrylamido) hexanoic acid)-grafted silica particles. *Polym. J.*, **43**, 778–784.

23. Fujii, S., Aono, K., Suzaki, M., Hamasaki, S., Yusa, S., and Nakamura, Y. (2012). pH-responsive hairy particles synthesized by dispersion polymerization with a macroinitiator as an inistab and their use as a gas-sensitive liquid marble stabilizer. *Macromolecules*, **45**(6), 2863–2873.

24. Nakai, K., Nakagawa, H., Kuroda, K., Fujii, S., Nakamura, Y., and Yusa, S. (2013). Near-infrared-responsive liquid marbles stabilized with carbon nanotubes. *Chem. Lett.*, **42**(7), 719–721.

25. Nakai, K., Fujii, S., Nakamura, Y., and Yusa, S. (2013). Ultraviolet light-responsive liquid marbles. *Chem. Lett.*, **42**(6), 586–588.

26. Yusa, S., Morihara, M., Nakai, K., Fujii, S., Nakamura, Y., Maruyama, A., and Shimada, N. (2014). Thermo-responsive liquid marbles. *Polym. J.*, **46**, 145–148.

27. Ueno, K., Hamasaki, S., Wanless, E. J., Nakamura, Y., and Fujii, S. (2014). Microcapsules fabricated from liquid marbles stabilized with latex particles. *Langmuir*, **30**(11), 3051–3059.

28. Ueno, K., Bournival, G., Wanless, E. J., Nakayama, S., Giakoumatos, E. C., Nakamura, Y., and Fujii, S. (2015). Liquid marble and water droplet interactions and stability. *Soft Matter*, **11**(39), 7728–7738.

29. Nakai, K., Fujii, S., Nakamura, Y., and Yusa, S. (2015). Thermoresponsive liquid marbles prepared with low melting point powder. *Chem. Lett.*, **44**(8), 1077–1079.

30. Kozuka, S., Banno, T., Fujii, S., Nakamura, Y., and Yusa, S. (2019). Disruption of liquid marbles induced by host-guest interaction. *Chem. Lett.*, **48**(8), 840–843.

31. Yukioka, S., Fujiwara, J., Okada, M., Fujii, S., Nakamura, Y., and Yusa, S. (2020). CO_2 gas-responsive liquid marble. *Langmuir*, **36**(25), 6971–6976.

32. Tian, J., Arbatan, T., Li, X., and Shen, W. (2010). Liquid marble for gas sensing, *Chem. Commun.*, **46**(26), 4734–4736.

33. Paven, M., Mayama, H., Sekido, T., Butt, H.-J., Nakamura, Y., and Fujii, S. (2016). Light-driven delivery and release of materials using liquid marbles. *Adv. Funct. Mater.*, **26**(19), 3199–3206.

34. Kawashima, H., Mayama, H., Nakamura, Y., and Fujii, S. (2017). Hydrophobic polypyrrole synthesized by aqueous chemical oxidative polymerization and its use as a light-responsive liquid marble stabilizer. *Polym. Chem.*, **8**(17), 2609–2618.

35. Kawashima, H., Paven, M., Mayama, H., Butt, H.-J., Nakamura, Y., and Fujii, S. (2017). Transfer of materials from water to solid surfaces by using liquid marbles. *ACS Appl. Mater. Interfaces*, **9**(38), 33351–33359.

36. Kawashima, H., Okatani, R., Mayama, H., Nakamura, Y., and Fujii, S. (2018). Synthesis of hydrophobic polyanilines as a light-responsive liquid marble stabilizer. *Polymer*, **148**, 217–227.

37. Shimogama, N., Uda, M., Oyama, K., Hanochi, H., Hirai, T., Nakamura, Y., and Fujii, S. (2019). Hydrophobic poly(3,4-ethylenedioxythiophene) particles synthesized by aqueous oxidative coupling polymerization and their use as near-infrared-responsive liquid marble stabilizer. *Polym. J.*, **51**, 761–770.

38. Inoue, H., Hirai, T., Hanochi, H., Oyama, K., Mayama, H., Nakamura, Y., and Fujii, S. (2019). Poly(3-hexylthiophene) grains synthesized by solvent-free oxidative coupling polymerization and their use as light-responsive liquid marble stabilizer. *Macromolecules*, **52**(2), 708–717.

39. Šišáková, M., Asaumi, Y., Uda, M., Seike, M., Oyama, K., Higashimoto, S., Hirai, T., Nakamura, Y., and Fujii, S. (2020). Dodecyl sulfate-doped polypyrrole derivative grains as a light-responsive liquid marble stabilizer. *Polym. J.*, **52**, 589–599.

40. Pike, N., Richard, D., Foster, W., and Mahadevan, L. (2002). How aphids lose their marbles. *Proc. R. Soc. B*, **269**(1497), 1211–1215.

41. Kasahara, M., Akimoto, S., Hariyama, T., Takaku, Y., Yusa, S., Okada, S., Nakajima, K., Hirai, T., Mayama, H., Okada, S., Deguchi, S., Nakamura, Y., and Fujii, S. (2019). Liquid marbles in nature: craft of aphids for survival. *Langmuir*, **35**(18), 6169–6178.

42. Aussillous, P., and Quéré, D. (2000). Liquid marbles. *Nature*, **411**, 924–927.

43. Klingauf, F. A. (1987). Feeding, adaptation and excretion, in *Aphid: Their Biology, Natural Enemies and Control*, Vol. 2A (Minks, A. K., and Harrewijn, P., eds), pp. 225–253.

44. Völkl, W., Woodring, J., Fischer, M., Lorenz, M. W., and Hoffmann, K. H. (1999). Ant-aphid mutualisms: the impact of honeydew production and honeydew sugar composition on ant preferences. *Oecologia*, **118**, 483–491.

45. Fischer, M. K., and Shingleton, A. W. (2001). Host plant and ants influence the honeydew sugar composition of aphids. *Funct. Ecol.*, **15**, 544–550.

46. Sasaki, T., Aoki, T., Hayashi, H., and Ishikawa, H. (1990). Amino acid composition of the honeydew of symbiotic and aposymbiotic pea aphids *Acyrthosiphon pisum. J. Insect Physiol.*, **36**, 35–40.

47. Leroy, P. D., Wathelet, B., Sabri, A., Francis, F., Verheggen, F. J., Capella, Q., Thonart, P., and Haubruge, E. (2011). Aphid-host plant interactions: does aphid honeydew exactly reflect the host plant amino acid composition? *Arthropod-Plant Inte.*, **5**, 193–199.

48. Yao, I., and Akimoto, S. (2002). Flexibility in the composition and concentration of amino acids in honeydew of the drepanosiphid aphid, *Tuberculatus quercicola. Ecol. Entomol.*, **27**, 745–752.

49. Woodring, J., Wiedemann, R., Fischer, M. K., Hoffmann, K. H., and Völkl, W. (2004). Honeydew amino acids in relation to sugars and their role in the establishment of ant attendance hierarchy in eight species of aphids feeding on tansy (*Tanacetum vulgare*). *Physiol. Entomol.*, **29**, 311–319.

50. Dixon, A. F. G. (1985). *Aphid Ecology An Optimization Approach*, Springer, Netherlands.

51. Akimoto, S. (1983). A revision of the genus eriosoma and its allied genera in Japan (Homoptera: Aphidoidea). *Insecta Matsumuran A*, **27**, 37–106.

52. Suzuki, D. K., Fukushi, Y., and Akimoto, S. (2009). Do aphid galls provide good nutrients for the aphids?: Comparisons of amino acid concentrations in galls among *Tetraneura* species (Aphididae: Eriosomatinae). *Arthropod-Plant Inte.*, **3**, 241–247.

53. Aoki, S. (1980). Occurrence of a simple labor in a gall aphid, pemphigus dorocola (Homoptera, Pemphigidae), *Kontyu*, **48**(1), 71–73.

Chapter 12

Fabrication of Artificial Melanin-Based Structural Color Materials through Biomimetic Design

Michinari Kohri

Graduate School of Engineering, Chiba University, 1-33 Yayoi-cho, Inage-ku, Chiba 263-8522, Japan

kohri@faculty.chiba-u.jp

12.1 Introduction

Natural colors are mainly classified into two types: pigment colors and structural colors. A pigment color is a remaining color that is visible by absorbing light of a specific wavelength. In contrast, a structural color is a color that appears when light hits a submicron-sized periodic structure. Familiar examples include soap bubbles and rainbow colors on a back of compact disc. In each case, there is no inherent color of materials. The former is a color derived from thin-film interference caused by the difference in the refractive index between the air and the thin film of the soap bubble, and the latter is a diffraction grating formed in fine irregularities on the surface. Pigment colors are easily discolored by the decomposition of dyes through ultraviolet

---

Biomimetics: Connecting Ecology and Engineering by Informatics
Edited by Akihiro Miyauchi and Masatsugu Shimomura
Copyright © 2023 Jenny Stanford Publishing Pte. Ltd.
ISBN 978-981-4968-10-2 (Hardcover), 978-1-003-27717-0 (eBook)
www.jennystanford.com

irradiation. On the other hand, a structural color does not fade as long as the structure is maintained. The most prominent example is the color of fossil bird feathers. Fossils formed by replacing tissue with minerals are usually colorless, but, very rarely, colored fossils have been found [1]. The color of these fossils has been reported to be a structural color due to the microstructure formed inside the wing feathers.

Colloidal crystals spontaneously form periodic microstructures which produce structural colors due to physical phenomena, such as light interference, diffraction, and scattering when exposed to light; there is no fading as long as the fine structure is maintained. Structural colors with unique lusters, high color development and durability are expected to be applied in various fields, and much research has been conducted. In designing colloidal crystals, materials and methods that form the microstructures are important.

This chapter introduces the fabrication of colloidal crystals using artificial melanin particles based on polydopamine and their use as a component of biomimetic structural color materials and research trends in peripheral fields.

12.2 Structural Colors Found in Nature

12.2.1 Role of Melanin in Structural Coloration

Structural colors are often found in bright colors of insects, fish, plants and animals. Typical examples include the coloring of *Morpho* butterflies, jewel beetles, and peacock feathers. Melanin is a brown to black substance that is well known as a component of human hair and skin. It has the function of protecting skin from ultraviolet rays, plays an important role in the structural color of these organisms. The color of the blue *Morpho* butterfly wing is derived from the shelf structure with a melanin layer below the shelf structure [2]. The color of a jewel beetle's wings is a structural color derived from a multilayer film in which a melanin layer and a cuticle layer are alternately laminated [3]. Inside peacock feathers, rod-shaped melanin granules form a regular microstructure, causing beautiful structural colors [4]. The size of these microstructures is on the order of hundreds of nanometers.

In general, when light hits these submicron-sized structures, the light appears white to the human eye due to light scattering. When part of the microstructure is formed by black melanin, it appears brighter to the human eye because the scattered light is absorbed and the structural color becomes more enhanced. In other words, in bright structural coloration in the natural world, melanin plays an important role in the construction of a fine structure and the suppression of scattered light.

12.2.2 Melanin and Polydopamine

In vivo, melanin is produced from dopa, an amino acid, by a complex reaction involving multistep enzymatic reactions [5]. For this reason, it is extremely difficult to perform artificial synthesis of melanin with the fine structural control required for the creation of structural colors using the biosynthetic pathway. Dopamine is one of the metabolites of dopa in vivo and is easily polymerized by self-oxidation in a basic solution to obtain polydopamine [6]. Polydopamine is widely used as a surface

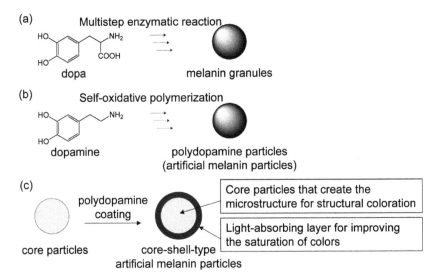

Figure 12.1 (a) Chemical structure of natural melanin and (b) polydopamine (artificial melanin), and (c) design of core–shell-type artificial melanin particles.

modifier because it adheres to various types of base-material surface. The structures of dopa and dopamine are similar, and from a chemical structural point of view, polydopamine is a material with almost the same composition as that of natural melanin and is regarded as easily prepared artificial melanin (Fig. 12.1a,b) [7].

12.3 Structural Coloration by Assembly of Colloidal Particles

Optical phenomena that produce structural colors include thin-film interference, multilayer interference, diffraction gratings, and scattering. The development of artificial structural color materials utilizing these properties is ongoing. Among them, much research has been conducted on structural color materials using colloidal crystals, which are assemblies of colloidal particles. A periodic structure in which monodisperse colloidal particles having a particle diameter of several hundred nm close to the wavelength of light and that are regularly arranged is called a colloidal crystal structure. It is known that the structural color of colloidal crystal structures conforms to the following Bragg–Snell equation (12.1) [8]:

$$m\lambda = \sqrt{\frac{8}{3}d^2(n^2 - \sin^2\theta)},$$ (12.1)

where m is the diffraction grating, λ is the light wavelength, d is the distance between particles, n is the refractive index of the colloidal particles, and θ is the auxiliary angle of the incident angle. The coloration, saturation, and angle dependencies of the structural colors produced from colloidal crystals are controlled by the particle size, refractive index, blackness, and assembled structure of the particles used. Based on these four parameters, research and development of artificial structural color materials are proceeding from various viewpoints [9].

12.4 Structural Color Materials from Artificial Melanin Particles

12.4.1 Structural Coloration from Polydopamine Particles

When dopamine is polymerized in a mixed water/methanol solvent, black polydopamine particles with relatively uniform particle sizes can be obtained [10]. By concentrating the obtained aqueous dispersion of submicron-sized polydopamine particles and constructing an assembled structure, a structural color corresponding to the particle diameter was observed (Fig. 12.2) [10]. Since polydopamine particles disperse well in water, structural coloration by spray painting was also possible. Following the structural coloration mechanism in nature, by creating an assembled structure with black particles of uniform size, light scattering was suppressed, and vivid structural coloration was realized by polydopamine particles. These colors are structural colors resulting from scattering that occurs due to the assembly of submicron-sized polydopamine particles. The dispersion properties of the particles can also be controlled by coating the surface of the polydopamine particles with a magnetic surfactant [11] or modifying the surface by constructing graft polymers by living polymerization [12].

Structural colors based on thin film interference using polydopamine particles have also been reported. Xiao et al. reported that polydopamine particles with a particle size of approximately 100 nm were used to form a thin film, and the structural color changed according to the film thickness [13]. In this case, the colors can be controlled by changing the thickness of the film using the hygroscopicity of polydopamine particles [14]. Furthermore, it has been reported by Wu et al. [15], Kawamura et al. [16], and Zhang et al. [17] that polydopamine can be colored by depositing polydopamine in the form of a thin film and not in the form of particles.

Particles prepared with only polydopamine, which is a light absorber, are very dark. Thus, the color of the obtained structural color materials becomes dark. To obtain a structural color, it is necessary to darken the surroundings and shine light on the particles with a strong light source. Cho et al. reported on the application of polydopamine particles as an anti-counterfeiting technology, utilizing the property that the structural color visibility of polydopamine particle-assemblies is different before and after light irradiation [18].

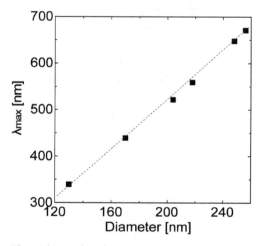

Figure 12.2 The relationship between polydopamine particle size and the reflection wavelength of the structural color materials.

12.4.2 Structural Coloration by Core–Shell Particles with Polydopamine as the Shell Layer

12.4.2.1 Particle design

Core–shell-type artificial melanin particles coated with polydopamine were designed and manufactured using monodisperse polystyrene core particles to adjust the degree of blackness and light absorption [19]. By changing the feed concentration of the dopamine monomer when forming the shell layer, a polydopamine shell layer with an arbitrary thickness was formed, and the blackness of the particles was easily controlled (Fig. 12.3). Monodisperse core particles are important for microstructural construction, and the black polydopamine shell layer is necessary for scattered light absorption.

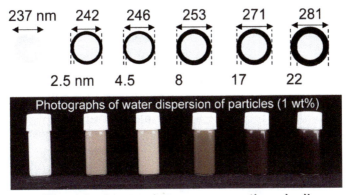

Figure 12.3 Shell thickness and blackness of core–shell-type artificial melanin particles.

12.4.2.2 High-visibility structural coloration

Polystyrene core particles are materials that have been conventionally used in the production of colloidal crystals. An aqueous dispersion of particles was dropped onto a silicone rubber, and solid pellet samples were prepared by a natural drying process. When polystyrene particles were used as a component, milky-white structural color pellets were obtained. In contrast, core–shell-type artificial melanin particles resulted in highly visible structural color pellets [19]. Figure 12.4 shows the reflectance spectra of the surfaces of pellets prepared from polystyrene particles and core–shell-type artificial melanin particles. While the reflectivity of the peak at approximately 480 nm due to the blue structural color was higher for pellets made of polystyrene particles than for pellets made of core–shell-type artificial melanin particles, the background due to light scattering was also higher throughout the visible light range. Thus, it looked white to the human eye (Fig. 12.4, dotted line). On the other hand, in the pellet made of the core–shell-type artificial melanin particles, the background was totally reduced (Fig. 12.4, solid line). The reflectance of the structural colors was also reduced, but the visibility to the human eye was dramatically improved because the light-absorbing layer made of polydopamine effectively absorbed scattered light.

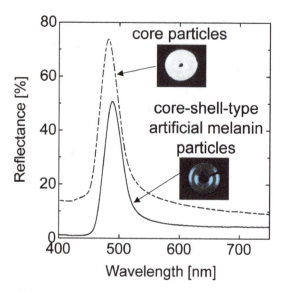

Figure 12.4 Reflectance measurement results of pellets obtained from polystyrene particles (dotted line) and core–shell-type artificial melanin particles (solid line). Insets show photographs of structural color pellets.

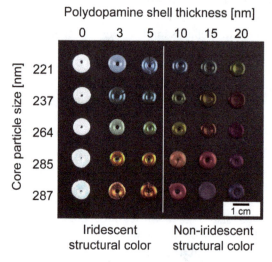

Figure 12.5 Structural color pellets produced by controlling the core particle size and polydopamine shell thickness.

When creating core–shell-type artificial melanin particles, almost all colors were obtained by controlling the core particle diameter and the thickness of the polydopamine shell layer (Fig. 12.5) [19]. Since the pellet shown in Fig. 12.5 was fabricated using only core–shell particles, the assembled structure was easily broken by external stress. For practical use, it is important to develop a technology to cure the colloidal crystal structure. It has been reported that silane coupling agents [20, 21], polyurethane particles [22], and alkali vapor treatment [23] can be used to cure assembled structures composed of core–shell particles made with polydopamine shells.

12.4.2.3 Effect of assembled structures on coloration

The colors of peacock feathers are iridescent structural colors, which are caused by the periodic structure of rod-shaped melanin granules, and the hue of the structural color changes depending on the viewing angle [4, 24]. In contrast, the blue feathers of *Cotinga maynana* are non-iridescent structural colors in which the same color is seen regardless of the viewing angle. An amorphous structure consisting of melanin granules and pigments formed inside the feathers of *Cotinga maynana* [25]. While the amorphous structure does not contain long-range order, the short-range order is maintained, and a non-iridescent structural color developed by selective reflection depending on the particle size [26].

Interestingly, for structural color pellets made by assembly of core–shell-type artificial melanin particles, the angular dependence of structural color can be easily controlled by the thickness of the polydopamine shell layer [19]. Particles with a shell layer thickness of less than 5 nm formed a colloidal crystal structure that exhibited an iridescent structural color (Figs. 12.5 and 12.6, left). In contrast, particles having a shell layer thickness of 10 nm or more exhibited a non-iridescent structural color due to the amorphous structure (Figs. 12.5 and 12.6, right). As the thickness of the polydopamine shell layer increased, the roughness of the particle surface increased, affecting the arrangement of particles. Controlling the angular dependence of structural colors is an important subject in practical use. In this method, control of the arrangement of particles and the angular dependence of structural colors can only be achieved by controlling the thickness of the polydopamine shell layer.

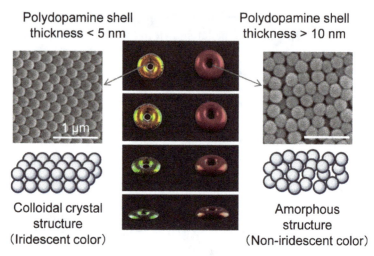

Figure 12.6 Difference in angle dependencies of structural color and difference in microstructure of material surface.

The angle dependence of the structural color was also controlled by particle mixing [27]. When artificial melanin particles of different sizes were mixed to form a pellet, the particle arrangement changed according to the mixing ratio, and the angle dependences of the structural colors changed. In this case, the average particle diameter of the particles can be adjusted stepwise by mixing the particles. The structural color depends on the particle diameter as shown in Eq. (12.1); therefore an intermediate structural color can be obtained by color adjustment using a mixing of the particles with various diameters, which is expected to be applied to various coloring systems.

12.4.2.4 Effect of compositions on coloration

Melanin is the black component of human hair, and individual hair- color varies from person to person. This is due to differences in melanin content and its composition. As mentioned above, an example was shown in which dopamine was used as a precursor monomer for producing core–shell-type artificial melanin. Instead of dopamine, artificial melanin particles are formed from dopamine and norepinephrine, which exist in the body before and after the metabolic pathway of dopamine (Fig. 12.7) [28].

Although oxidizing reagents were required to accelerate the polymerization, core–shell particles could be prepared using dopa and norepinephrine, resulting in highly visible structural colors. In particular, it was found that the surface of core–shell particle using norepinephrine became smoother than that of using dopamine or dopa. As a result, structural colors with angle dependence were easily obtained by using norepinephrine. Furthermore, the properties of the produced artificial melanin particles changed with the type of melanin precursor-monomer, and the resulting structural color was also affected.

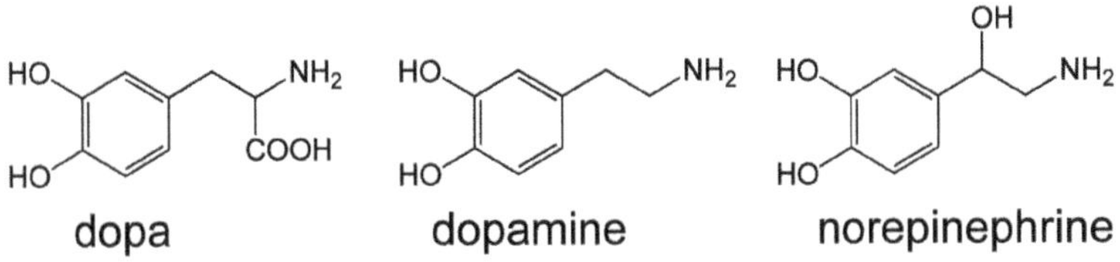

dopa   dopamine   norepinephrine

Figure 12.7 Chemical structures of melanin precursor monomers.

12.4.2.5 Effect of particle shapes on coloration

Generally, spherical and solid particles are used as a component of structural color materials formed by the assembly of colloidal particles. However, looking at the natural world, particle shapes vary widely. In the case of peacock feathers, rod-shaped melanin granules [4, 24] are used as a component for constructing a microstructure, and hollow melanin granules are used in turkeys [29]. It is considered that the shapes of these constituents affect the structural coloration.

When a polyvinyl alcohol film containing core–shell-type artificial melanin particles was extended under heating and melted after cooling, then ellipsoidal artificial melanin particles were obtained. The aspect ratio of particle was controlled by the stretch ratio of the film containing the particles (Fig. 12.8a). The minor axis length of the ellipsoidal particles affected the structural color, and the continuous structural color blueshifted with increasing aspect ratio (Fig. 12.8b) [30]. This is because ellipsoidal artificial melanin particles were likely to be deposited laterally on the substrate.

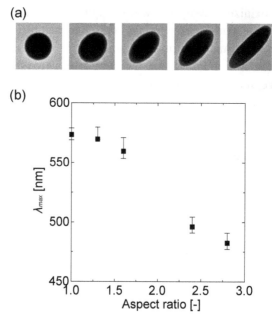

Figure 12.8 (a) Transmission electron microscope images of core–shell-type artificial melanin particles with different aspect ratios and (b) the relationship between the particle aspect ratio and reflection wavelength.

Multiple coatings of a polydopamine shell layer resulted in robust core–shell-type artificial melanin particles with a thick shell. When the core particles were dissolved by solvent treatment, hollow artificial melanin particles were obtained. According to Eq. (12.1), the wavelength of the structural color is highly dependent on the refractive index of the material. Hollow particles have a different refractive index than that of solid particles. This is because the internal voids form spaces and the structural color tone changes significantly [28].

12.4.2.6 Application as coloring materials

In developing an ink colorant based on a structural color, the background color is important for observing the structural color. If a white background, such as paper, is used to observe the structural color, light scattering reduces the visibility of the structural color. Thus, a black background is often used to improve the visibility of structural colors. Since artificial melanin particles, which are black particles, have light absorbing ability, structural colors with high visibility were observed even when using a white background as well as a black background [31]. This feature will be a great advantage for their use as a colorant in inks.

Core–shell-type artificial melanin particles were well dispersed in aqueous media due to their high zeta potential (approximately –50 mV) [19]. Taking advantage of this feature, structural color printing has been performed by an inkjet method using an aqueous dispersion of artificial melanin particles as ink [32]. It was observed that after inkjet printing, a dome-shaped structure composed of particle-assembles were formed in the sample. Structural color inkjet printing of each color was possible depending on the size of the particles used (Fig. 12.9). Furthermore, using the membrane emulsification method, W/O emulsions containing artificial melanin particles were obtained. Spherical structural color materials were formed by heating this emulsion (Fig. 12.10a) [33]. Continuous production of W/O emulsions using microchannels resulted in fibrous structural color materials (Fig. 12.10b) [33]. Using these three-dimensional structural color materials as constituent units, the development of new coloring materials will be expected to replace conventional dyes and pigments.

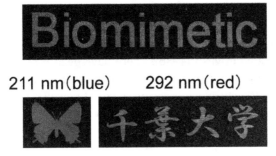

Figure 12.9 Structural color prints by the inkjet method using core–shell-type artificial melanin particles as ink.

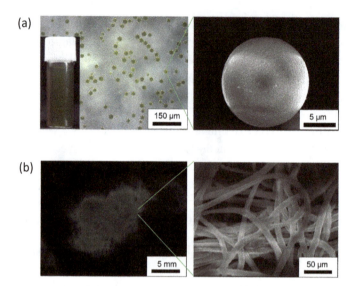

Figure 12.10 (a) Spherical and (b) fibrous structural color materials based on a W/O emulsion containing core–shell-type artificial melanin particles.

12.5 Structural Coloration by Black Additives

The previous section described structural color materials obtained by assembly of black particles using polydopamine as a component. In this method, the black particles can be used as a single component and can represent bright structural colors. On the other hand, adding a black substance to conventional systems that use polystyrene or silica particles also increases the color saturation of the structural color and improves the visibility of the structural color. Carbon blacks are commonly used as black additives [34–36]. There have been reports of using polypyrrole [37] or squid ink [38] as another black substance. While bright structural colors using the existing colloidal materials are necessary to mix the components properly.

12.6 Perspectives

Artificial melanin particles using polydopamine have been produced by mimicking natural melanin, which is important for structural coloration in nature. By using artificial melanin particles, which are black particles, the reflection and absorption of light were controlled, and bright and highly visible structural coloration was achieved by single colloidal material [39, 40]. In addition to its use as a colorant for inks, the development of cosmetics for the skin is also expected, since polydopamine is a highly biocompatible material prepared using materials that exist in the living body. While the usefulness of structural color materials using artificial melanin particles has been demonstrated, the mechanism by which periodic structures composed of melanin are formed in vivo is still unknown. Polydopamine is a material that mimics natural melanin, both in composition and structure, and is easy to create including microstructural control. In the future, the findings obtained in this research are expected to contribute to the progress of basic research to understand structural colors in nature, in addition to research for practical use.

Acknowledgments

This work was supported by a Grant-in-Aid for Scientific Research (B) (JSPS KAKENHI Grant Number: 17H03110) and Scientific Research on Innovative Areas "Engineering Neo-Biomimetics" (JSPS KAKENHI Grant Number: 15H01593).

References

1. Vinther, J., Briggs, D. E., Clarke, J., Mayr, G., and Prum, R. O. (2010). Structural coloration in a fossil feather. *Biol. Lett.*, **6**, 128–131.
2. Kinoshita, S., Yoshioka, S., Fujii, Y., and Okamoto, N. (2002). Photophysics of structural color in the *Morpho* butterflies. *Forma*, **17**, 103–121.
3. Yoshioka, S., Kinoshita, S., Iida, H., and Hariyama, T. (2012). Phase-adjusting layers in the multilayer reflector of a jewel beetle. *J. Phys. Soc. Jpn.*, **81**, 054801.
4. Yoshioka, S., and Kinoshita, S. (2002). Effect of macroscopic structure in iridescent color of the peacock feathers. *Forma*, **17**, 169–181.
5. Riley, P. A. (1997). Melanin. *Int. J. Biochem. Cell Biol.*, **29**, 1235–1239.
6. Lee, H., Dellatore, S. M., Miller, W. M., and Messersmith, P. B. (2007). Mussel-inspired surface chemistry for multifunctional coatings. *Science*, **318**, 426–430.

7. d'Ischia, M., Napolitano, A., Ball, V., Chen, C. T., and Buehler, M. J. (2014). Polydopamine and eumelanin: from structure-property relationships to a unified tailoring strategy. *Acc. Chem. Res.*, **47**, 3541–3550.

8. Ge, J., and Yin, Y. (2011). Responsive photonic crystals. *Angew. Chem. Int. Ed.*, **50**, 1492–1522.

9. Goerlitzer, E. S. A., Taylor, R. N. K., and Vogel, N. (2018). Bioinspired photonic pigments from colloidal self-assembly. *Adv. Mater.*, **30**, 1706654.

10. Kohri, M., Nannichi, Y., Taniguchi, T., and Kishikawa, K. (2015). Biomimetic non-iridescent structural color materials from polydopamine black particles that mimic melanin granules. *J. Mater. Chem. C.*, **3**, 720–724.

11. Kawamura, A., Kohri, M., Taniguchi, T., and Kishikawa, K. (2016). Surface modification of polydopamine particles *via* magnetically-responsive surfactants. *Trans. Mat. Res. Soc. Jpn.*, **41**, 301–304.

12. Kohri, M., Uradokoro, K., Nannichi, Y., Kawamura, A., Taniguchi, T., and Kishikawa, K. (2018). Hairy polydopamine particles as platforms for photonic and magnetic materials. *Photonics*, **5**, 36.

13. Xiao, M., Li, Y., Allen, M. C., Deheyn, D. D., Yue, X., Zhao, J., Gianneschi, N. C., Shawkey, M. D., and Dhinojwala, A. (2015). Bio-inspired structural colors produced *via* self-assembly of synthetic melanin nanoparticles. *ACS Nano*, **9**, 5454–5460.

14. Xiao, M., Li, Y., Zhao, J., Wang, Z., Gao, M., Gianneschi, N. C., Dhinojwala, A., and Shawkey, M. D. (2016). Stimuli-responsive structurally colored films from bioinspired synthetic melanin nanoparticles. *Chem. Mater.*, **28**, 5516–5521.

15. Wu, T. F., and Hong, J. D. (2015). Dopamine-melanin nanofilms for biomimetic structural coloration. *Biomacromolecules*, **16**, 660–666.

16. Kawamura, A., Kohri, M., Oku, H., Hamada, K., Nakagawa, K., Taniguchi, T., and Kishikawa, K. (2017). Structural color materials from polydopamine-inorganic hybrid thin films inspired by rock pigeon feathers. *Kobunshi Ronbunshu*, **74**, 54–58.

17. Zhang, C., Wu, B. H., Du, Y., Ma, M. Q., and Xu, Z. K. (2017). Mussel-inspired polydopamine coatings for large-scale and angle-independent structural colors. *J. Mater. Chem. C.*, **5**, 3898–3902.

18. Cho, S., Shim, T. S., Kim, J. H., Kim, D. H., and Kim, S. H. (2017). Selective coloration of melanin nanospheres through resonant mie scattering. *Adv. Mater.*, **29**, 1700256.

19. Kawamura, A., Kohri, M., Morimoto, G., Nannichi, Y., Taniguchi, T., and Kishikawa, K. (2016). Full-color biomimetic photonic materials with iridescent and non-iridescent structural colors. *Sci. Rep.*, **6**, 33984.

20. Yi, B., and Shen, H. (2017). Facile fabrication of crack-free photonic crystals with enhanced color contrast and low angle dependence. *J. Mater. Chem. C*, **5**, 8194–8200.

21. Yi, B., and Shen, H. (2018). Structurally colored films with superhydrophobicity and wide viewing angles based on bumpy melanin-like particles. *Appl. Surf. Sci.*, **427**, 1129–1136.

22. Chen, G., Yi, B., Huang, Y., Liang, Q., and Shen, H. (2019). Development of bright and low angle dependence structural colors from order-disorder hierarchical photonic structure. *Dyes Pigments*, **161**, 464–469.

23. Liu, P., Chen, J., Zhang, Z., Xie, Z., Du, X., and Gu, Z. (2018). Bio-inspired robust non-iridescent structural color with self-adhesive amorphous colloidal particle arrays. *Nanoscale*, **10**, 3673–3679.

24. Zi, J., Yu, X., Li, Y., Hu, X., Xu, C., Wang, X., Liu, X., and Fu, R. (2003). Coloration strategies in peacock feathers. *Proc. Natl. Acad. Sci. USA*, **100**, 12576.

25. Prum, R. O., Torres, R., Williamson, S., and Dyck, J. (1998). Coherent light scattering by blue feather barbs. *Nature*, **396**, 28–29.

26. Takeoka, Y. (2012). Angle-independent structural coloured amorphous arrays. *J. Mater. Chem.*, **22**, 23299–23309.

27. Kawamura, A., Kohri, M., Yoshioka, S., Taniguchi, T., and Kishikawa, K. (2017). Structural color tuning: mixing melanin-like particles with different diameters to create neutral colors. *Langmuir*, **33**, 3824–3830.

28. Iwasaki, T., Tamai, Y., Yamamoto, M., Taniguchi, T., Kishikawa, K., and Kohri, M. (2018). Melanin precursor influence on structural colors from artificial melanin particles: polyDOPA, polydopamine, and polynorepinephrine. *Langmuir*, **34**, 11814–11821.

29. Shawkey, M. D., D'Alba, L., Xiao, M., Schutte, M., and Buchholz, R. (2015). Ontogeny of an iridescent nanostructure composed of hollow melanosomes. *J. Morphol.*, **276**, 378–384.

30. Kohri, M., Tamai, Y., Kawamura, A., Jido, K., Yamamoto, M., Taniguchi, T., Kishikawa, K., Fujii, S., Teramoto, N., Ishii, H., and Nagao, D. (2019). Ellipsoidal artificial melanin particles as building blocks for biomimetic structural coloration. *Langmuir*, **35**, 5574–5580.

31. Kohri, M., Yamazaki, S., Kawamura, A., Taniguchi, T., and Kishikawa, K. (2017). Bright structural color films independent of background prepared by the dip-coating of biomimetic melanin-like particles having polydopamine shell layers. *Colloids Surf. A*, **532**, 564–569.

32. Kohri, M., and Kawamura, A. US patent 5/246,029.

33. Kohri, M., Yanagimoto, K., Kawamura, A., Hamada, K., Imai, Y., Watanabe, T., Ono, T., Taniguchi, T., and Kishikawa, K. (2018). Polydopamine-based 3D colloidal photonic materials: structural color balls and fibers from melanin-like particles with polydopamine shell layers. *ACS Appl. Mater. Interfaces*, **10**, 7640–7648.

34. Forster, J. D., Noh, H., Liew, S. F., Saranathan, V., Schreck, C. F., Yang, L., Park, J. G., Prum, R. O., Mochrie, S. G. J., O'Hern, C. S., Cao, H., and Dufresne, E. R. (2010). Biomimetic isotropic nanostructures for structural coloration. *Adv. Mater.*, **22**, 2939–2944.

35. Takeoka, Y., Yoshioka, S., Takano, A., Arai, S., Nueangnoraj, K., Nishihara, H., Teshima, M., Ohtsuka, Y., and Seki, T. (2013). Production of colored pigments with amorphous arrays of black and white colloidal particles, *Angew. Chem. Int. Ed.*, **252**, 7261–7265.

36. Takeoka, Y. (2018). Environment and human friendly colored materials prepared using black and white components. *Chem. Commun.*, **54**, 4905–4914.

37. Yang, X., Ge, D., Wu, G., Liao, Z., and Yang, S. (2016). Production of structural colors with high contrast and wide viewing angles from assemblies of polypyrrole black coated polystyrene nanoparticles. *ACS Appl. Mater. Interfaces*, **8**, 16289–16295.

38. Zhang, Y., Dong, B., Chen, A., Liu, X., Shi, L., and Zi, J. (2015). Using cuttlefish ink as an additive to produce non-iridescent structural colors of high color visibility. *Adv. Mater.*, **27**, 4719–4724.

39. Kohri, M. (2017). Structural color materials from melanin-like particles through biomimetic approach. *Acc. Mater. Surf. Res.*, **2**, 72–80.

40. Kohri, M. (2019). Artificial melanin particles: new building blocks for biomimetic structural coloration. *Polym. J.*, **51**, 1127–1135.

Chapter 13

Study of Bile Duct Stent Having Antifouling Properties Using Biomimetics Technique

Atsushi Sekiguchi

Litho Tech Japan Corporation, 2-6-6 Namiki, Kawaguchi, Saitama 332-0034, Japan

sekiguchi-pdg@ltj.co.jp

Biomimetics is a field of technologies based on imitating the functions and properties found in living organisms. The application of the super-water-repellent fine structure of lotus leaves to create waterproof products is a well-known example of biomimetics. The present study examined the surface structure of snail shells, which exhibit oleophobic property, namely oil repellency, and explored the feasibility of recreating this structure on the inner surfaces of conventional biliary stents. Observations of snail shells under an electron microscope show a covering of extremely fine protrusions of around 200 nm in size. When water enters the pores between these fine protrusions, a film of water exhibiting super-hydrophilic structure forms on the shell. Because water and oil are immiscible, this film repels oil. We would expect a stent-occlusion to be less likely with a biliary stent having this structure on its inner surface.

Biomimetics: Connecting Ecology and Engineering by Informatics
Edited by Akihiro Miyauchi and Masatsugu Shimomura
Copyright © 2023 Jenny Stanford Publishing Pte. Ltd.
ISBN 978-981-4968-10-2 (Hardcover), 978-1-003-27717-0 (eBook)
www.jennystanford.com

A biliary stricture caused by bile duct cancer or bile duct obstruction leads to icterus and may, in serious cases, induce a fatal hepatic failure. A surgical procedure that places indwelling biliary-stents inside makes the biliary-tract secure a passage of a bile flow. However, conventional stents are prone to occlusion due to the accumulation of biliary sludge, resulting in the need for a second surgery to replace the stent. This problem is attributable to the polyethylene used to make the biliary stents; polyethylene is susceptible to the adhesion of cholesterol and fats found in the bile, eventually leading to stent-occlusions. This chapter reports our efforts to develop biliary stents that feature antifouling properties inspired by biomimetics to address this problem; specifically, the development of oleophobic inner stent surfaces featuring super-hydrophilic structures inspired by snail shell surfaces.

13.1 Introduction

A flow of bile from a gallbladder to a duodenum is obstructed by a biliary stricture caused by bile duct cancer [1] or bile duct obstruction. When this occurs, the bile flows back into a liver, resulting in icterus. This condition leads to a hepatic failure, a potentially life-threatening condition, if left untreated. The condition is surgically treated by implanting an endoscopic biliary stent (EBS) [2, 3] as shown in Fig. 13.1.

Two types of biliary stent are currently available; metallic stents and plastic stents [4]. Plastic stents are generally used as EBSs. Figure 13.2 is a photograph of a straight plastic stent (PS). Each end has flaps and there is an opening beneath of each flap.

As is well known, a bile sludge tends to be collected in the stent because a bile is a viscous fluid containing fatty components such as cholesterol; resulting a stent-occlusion. To date, investigations seeking to prevent stent-occlusion have failed to get an adequate solution. In most cases, the problem is removing and replacing of stent in a second procedure [2]; undergoing multiple surgeries places significant stress on a patient. Developing a method to suppress the occlusion of biliary stents would reduce the number of surgeries per patient, which reduces burdens not just for the patient, but for clinical practitioners, including doctors. Therefore, the method and technical development are desired for suppressing an occlusion of biliary stents.

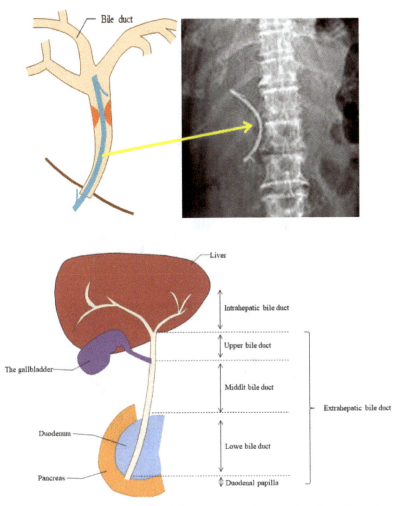

Figure 13.1 Structure of the biliary tract and example of endoscopic biliary stenting.

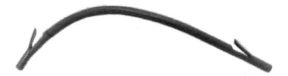

Figure 13.2 Plastic stent (straight type, Boston Scientific Corporation).

13.2 Biomimetics Technologies

As the observation of *"There are no dirty snails"* suggests that snail shells have superior antifouling performance. The snails during the *"baiu,"* a rainy season in Japan, always have clean and shining shells.

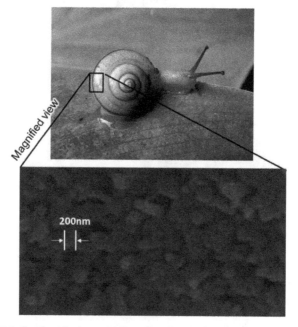

Figure 13.3 Snail with clean shell surface during *baiu*, a rainy season.

Snail shells are known to have convex-concave structures in nanoscale on their surface; approximately 200–400 nm (Fig. 13.3) that promote the formation of a water film on the shell surface, creating a super-hydrophilic structure that repels oils and stains

[5]. This super-hydrophilic structure has properties to repel oils containing proteins, etc. Figure 13.4 shows a schematic diagram of this principle. It should be possible to produce a super-hydrophilic structure by creating a structure mimicking the shell structure of snails. Here, the field of technologies based on mimicking various properties and structures observed in living organisms in nature is called biomimetics [6].

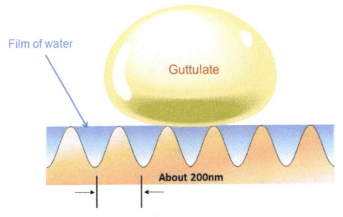

Figure 13.4 Super-hydrophilic effects of the nanoscale structure of snail shells.

The structure of the snail shell was observed in detail. Figure 13.5 is an SEM images of the snail shell. The snail shell has structures like a craggy mountain; surface scale of 20–40 μm. An enlarged view of the surface shows that these structures are formed by grains approximately 200 nm in size, and still further shows nanoscale holes between the grains.

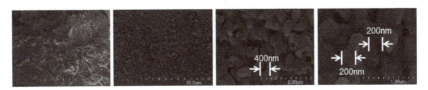

Figure 13.5 Snail shell structure (SEM image, top view).

Figure 13.6 shows the oil repellency on a Si substrate and snail shell in water. The contact-angle meter (model PAC-11 manufactured by Kyowa Interface Science Co., Ltd.) was modified for water observations. A sample is placed in water, and then an oil droplet is pressed out from the tip of a syringe needle, and contacts with the sample surface observing what happens; whether the oil droplet is repelled or adheres to the surface [7, 8]. In case of Si substrate, the droplet was found to adhere to the Si substrate (oil stain). However, the oil droplet was repelled from the snail shell, which exhibited oil repellency in water.

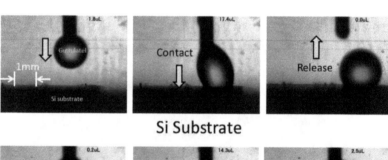

Si Substrate

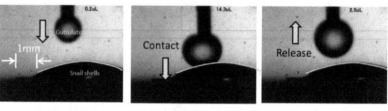

Shell of the snail

Figure 13.6 Oil repellency of snail shells: top, Si substrate; bottom, Shell of snail.

13.3 Biliary Stents with Antifouling Properties

An occluded biliary stent must be surgically replaced, typically endoscopically rather than by open surgery. If conditions contraindicate an endoscopic surgery, the alternatives are percutaneous transhepatic biliary drainage (PTBD) [9], in which the biliary tract is approached percutaneously (through the skin), or open surgery. However, repeated stent replacement procedures can be extremely stressful for the patient. A potential solution is fabricating an oleophobic fine structure of snail shells on the inner walls of biliary stents.

Regarding biomimetics productions, lotus leaves are a well-known example of super-water-repellency [6]. Inspired by the structures observed on these leaves, Nissan Motor Company is currently performing studies to produce super-water-repellent glass for automobiles. Such glass would remain free of water and ensure continuous clear views. Conventionally, fluorine-based hydrophobic coatings are applied to automobile glass for the same purpose. However, these coatings inevitably peel off with time, and the glass loses its water repellency. It has been explored that water repellent structures would achieve permanent hydrophobicity. However, such a technology does not repel oil. Bile, a fluid secreted by the liver, assists in the digestion and absorption of lipids by activating the digestive enzyme (lipase) to facilitate the dissolution of oil in water. The main constituents of bile are bilirubin, an end product of red-blood cell breakdown, cholesterol, and bile acid [10]. Bile is temporarily stored in the gallbladder before being excreted from the duodenum. In cases like the one above in which oleophobic properties would be beneficial, the structure of the snail shell, which exhibits super-hydrophilic effects in the presence of water, may help fabricate an occlusion-resistant biliary stent.

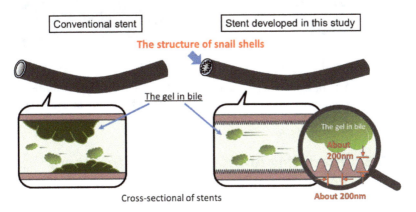

Figure 13.7 Comparison of conventional stent and antifouling stent (schematic image).

13.4 Production of Mold with Nanohole Structures Based on Snail Shell Surface Structures

To fabricate nanoscale structures inspired by snail shells, we formed 200 nm nano-holes on Si substrate by electron beam lithography. An electron beam resist (ZEP-520 positive tone resist: Zeon Corporation) of 300 nm was spin-coated onto Si substrate and baked; then electron beam lithography was performed using a mask design with an electron beam lithography unit. Then the resist was developed and etched the mold to create 200 nm nano-hole patterns on the Si substrate. Figure 13.8 shows the design of the lithographic pattern created for electron beam exposure and the SEM image of the nano-hole patterned on the Si mold. We obtained the mold with nano-holes of 200 nm diameter and 200 nm depth.

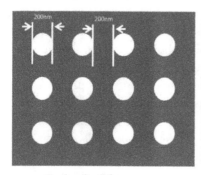
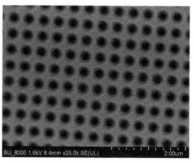

Design for EB exposure   SEM photo of Si nano-pattern mold

Figure 13.8 Design for electron beam (EB) exposure for 200 nm nano-hole patterns (left) and the formed nano-holes on Si mold by dry etching (right).

13.5 Producing Antifouling Sheets for Stents

Using the obtained mold with nano-scale structure and nanoimprint technology, we transferred the structure onto UV-curable acrylic polymers [11, 12]. The nanoimprinting method is described as follows. UV-curable acrylic polymer [13] was dropped onto a substrate (PET film); then the mold was pressed down onto the polymer. UV light is irradiated through the substrate from back-side as shown in Fig. 13.9. The LTNIP-5000 (Litho Tech Japan Corporation) was used as nanoimprinting machine [14]. The stamping pressure, UV light (365–436 nm) intensity, and exposure time were 1 kN, 7 mW/cm^2, and 5 min, respectively.

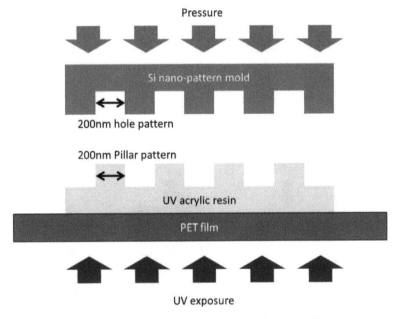

Figure 13.9 Schematic diagram of pattern transfer; nano-hole structure of the Si mold to the UV acrylic resin by UV nanoimprinting method.

Figure 13.10 shows a photograph of the pattern-transferred film and SEM images of formed patterns. The formation of 200 nm nano-pillar patterns on the PET film surface was confirmed by SEM observations. It was confirmed that both the nanostructured mold and polymer film exhibited oil repellency in water as shown in Fig. 13.11.

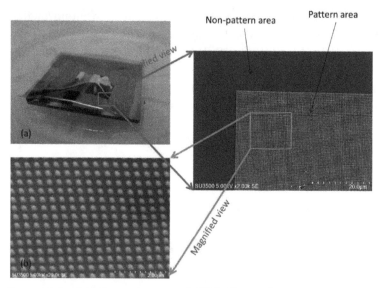

Figure 13.10 (a) External view of PET film with transferred nanostructure; (b) SEM image.

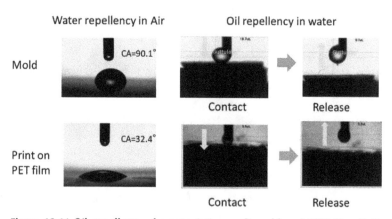

Figure 13.11 Oil repellency characteristics on Si mold and PET film. Both surface have nanostructure.

13.6 Fabrication of Biliary Stent and Liquid Passage Test

The nanoimprinted polymer sheet with antifouling properties was rolled to form a tube and placed inside a biliary stent.

Figure 13.12 shows the illustrations of how we produced the biliary stent and photographs of the finished products. The iridescent region is the part with the biomimetic structure. We passed an artificial bile solution consisting of a mixture of bovine bile and oil through the finished biliary stent to observe the manner of the liquid passage. The artificial bile solution was prepared by dissolving a powder of bovine bile in pure water to achieve a concentration of 10 wt.%; adding lard to this solution at a concentration of 10 wt.%; then heating to 40°C.

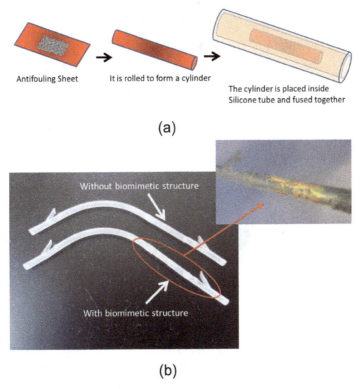

Figure 13.12 Illustration of method for producing biliary stent with antifouling properties (a) and photographs of the finished product (b).

Figure 13.13 gives an external view of the apparatus for the liquid passage evaluation. In the liquid passage test, the artificial bile solution was passed through the tube with a pump and the passage of the liquid observed in the part with the biomimetic structure.

290 | *Study of Bile Duct Stent Having Antifouling Properties Using Biomimetics Technique*

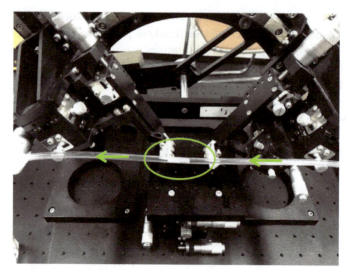

Figure 13.13 Apparatus for liquid passage evaluations; the region with biomimetic structure is indicated by a circle.

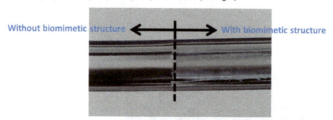

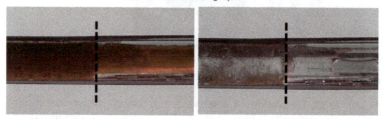

Figure 13.14 Results of liquid passage test using liquid mixture of bile and oil (lard).

After the passage of the bile-oil mixture, as shown in Fig. 13.14, the inner surface without the biomimetic structure showed oil adhesion. However, the part of the tube with the structure showed oil repellency. These findings suggest that oil repellency structure formed by nanoimprinting is expected for a highly oleophobic biliary stent.

13.7 In vivo Study

We placed indwelling biliary stents based on the biomimetic structure in the bile ducts of pigs and made SEM observations of the resulting stent conditions.

13.7.1 Overview of in vivo Study

The animals used in the study were female pigs (N = 2 animals, 20–30 kg). All were fasted preoperatively for 12 h (Category C). All procedures were performed under general anesthesia with mechanical ventilation, induced by intramuscular (IM) administration of ketamine hydrochloride (10 mg/kg) and atropine sulfate (IM, 0.05 mg/kg) administered as a preanesthetic to suppress tracheal and salivary secretions before endotracheal intubation. General anesthesia was maintained with sevoflurene (2–3%) inspiration and Musculax (0.5 mg/kg).

13.7.2 In vivo Study Procedure

After transportation, the pigs were acclimatized with a period of regular diet. To place the stents, we restricted the pigs to a supine position, then accessed the intraperitoneal cavity with an upper-abdominal median incision, by the method described in the above reference to reduce suffering. After exposing the common bile duct and duodenum, we made an incision to open the anterior duodenum wall, located the duodenal papilla, and inserted the biliary stent tube being evaluated through it to deliver the stent from the common bile duct into the duodenum. The stent was thereafter fixed to the duodenum wall using 4-0 PDS (0.15 mm absorbable synthetic monofilament). We used the 4-0 PDS to suture and close the duodenum wall after completing the stent implant procedure (Category D). The pigs were started on a liquid diet one day after this procedure and were switched to regular diet three days after this procedure, taking into consideration of the observations on their general condition. Seven days after the operation, the pigs were euthanized and their intraperitoneal cavities reopened to retrieve the stent. Euthanasia was performed via intravenous administration of ketamine hydrochloride (20 mg/kg).

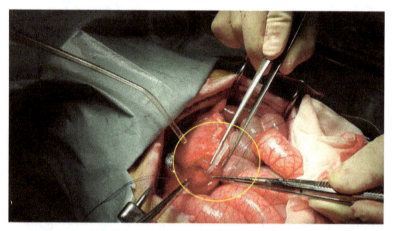

Figure 13.15 Surgical procedure for inserting biliary stent into the bile duct of a pig.

13.7.3 Results of Animal Testing (Antifouling Evaluations)

We evaluated the antifouling effect by visual and electron microscope observations of the regions with and without the biomimetic structure in the biliary stents. Visual observations with the unaided eye showed less fouling on the surface with biomimetic structures than without one as shown in Fig. 13.16. Furthermore, a clear difference in extent of fouling between regions with and without the biomimetic structure was confirmed by electron microscope observations as shown in Fig. 13.17. Table 13.1 is the quantitative results of antifouling obtained by SEM observations. The results indicate the antifouling performance of surfaces that feature the biomimetic structure is 58–85% better than surfaces without the structure.

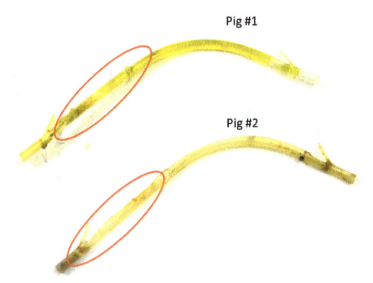

Figure 13.16 Biliary stents removed after indwelling for one week in bile duct of pigs (Pig #1 and #2; regions with biomimetic structure are circled in red.).

Table 13.1 Summary of antifouling effects

Pig No.	Structure	Fouled surface area (μm^2)	Mean fouling rate (%) *1
Pig #1	With structure 1	96.9	7.6
	With structure 2	89.6	
	With structure 3	101	
Pig #1	Without structure 1	675.1	49.5
	Without structure 2	597.1	
	Without structure 3	596.7	
Pig #2	With structure 1	393.7	23.9
	With structure 2	211	
	With structure 3	296.8	
Pig #2	Without structure 1	665.9	57.4
	Without structure 2	707.9	
	Without structure 3	795	

Total surface area of observed region 1,260 (μm^2).

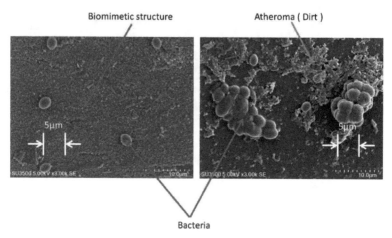

Figure 13.17 Results of SEM observations of biliary stents removed after indwelling for one week in bile duct of pig.

Mean fouling rate (%) = 100 × (fouled surface area/total surface area of observed region).

13.8 Summary

We produced a polymer film with antifouling properties by replicating a biomimetic structure on a polymer surface. We rolled the flat polymer sheet into a tube for use in biliary stents. These stents were implanted in the bile ducts of pigs to examine antifouling performance. The results show the polymer sheets are suitable for use in biliary stents and exhibit strong antifouling properties. Future studies will address mold production and stent manufacturing methods suitable for mass production.

Acknowledgments

We wish to express our gratitude to Mr. Shigeru Shimizu and Mr. Kazumi Chida at Photosensitive Materials Research Center of the Toyo Gosei Co., Ltd., for providing the UV-curable polymer (PAK-01) used in this study. We would also like to thank Ms. Natsuko Nagamatsu at the Nanotechnology Hub in Kyoto University for her contributions to the FE-SEM observation.

We thank Mr. Hiroshi Machida at Saitama Industrial Promotion Public Corporation for his technical guidance. This research was supported by the New Technology Products Realization and Development Grants Project of Saitama Prefecture for FY2017.

References

1. Masselli G, Manfredi R, Vecchioli A, Gualdi G, MR imaging and MR cholangiopancreatography in the preoperative evaluation of hilar cholangiocarcinoma: correlation with surgical and pathologic findings. *Eur Radiol* 2008; **18**, 2213–2221.

2. Tsuyuguchi T, Takada T, Kawarada Y, Nimura Y, Wada K, Nagino M, et al. Techniques of biliary drainage for acute cholangitis: Tokyo Guidelines. *J Hepatobiliary Pancreat Surg* 2007; **14**, 35–45.

3. http://www.shimadahp.jp/section.php?x-vew=4&from=section&nav i=3&sin=6, By Shimada hospital HP.

4. Smith AC, Dowsett JF, Rassell RC, Hartfield AR, Cotton PB, Randomized trial of endoscopic stenting versus surgical bypass in malignant low bileduct obstruction. Lancet 1994; **344**, 1655–1660.

5. Shimomura M, *Biomimetics, National Science Museum16*, Tokai University Press, 2, 2016.

6. Knippers J, Nickel KG, Speck T, *Biomimetic Research for Architecture and Building Construction, Biological Design and Integrative Structures*, *Biologically Inspired System* vol. 9, Springer, 69, 2016.

7. Kato M, Contact angle measurement with a microdroplet discharged by the Ink-Jet Head. *Journal of Printing Science and Technology* 2011; **48**(3), 186–190.

8. Kimura J, Itoh T, Koishi M, The measurements of contact angles of teflon powder and the consideration of the dependency of tablet porosity for the wetting. *Journal of Japan Society of Colour Material* UDC 532, 1977; **64**, 431–439.

9. Hirano S, Tanaka E, Tsuchikawa T, Matsumoto J, Kawakami H, Nakamura T, et al. Oncological benefit of preoperative endoscopic drainage in parietns with hilar cholangiocarcinoma. *J Hepatogiliary Pancreat Sci* 2014; **21**, 533–540.

10. Hajime T, Bile, Basic and clinical aspects of bile acids. *JJBA* 2011; **25**, 189–195.

11. Hiroshi Hiroshima, Nanoimprint with thin and uniform residual layer for various pattern densities. *Microelectron En* 2009; **86**(4–6), 611.

12. Hiroshima H, Atobe H, Homogeneity of residual layer thickness in UV nanoimprint lithography. *Jpn J Appl Phys* 2009; **48**, 06FH18.

13. Sakai N, Hirasawa T, Photo-curable resine for UV nanoimprint and their evaluation methods. *The Society of Polymer Science Japan* 2009; **66**, 88–96.

14. Sekiguchi A, Kono Y, Hirai Y, Study on polymer materials evaluation system for nano-imprint lithography. *J Photopolymer* 2004; **16**, 463.

Chapter 14

Biomimetic Designed Surfaces for Growth Suppression of Biofilm-Inspired Sharkskin Denticles

Mariko Miyazaki[a] and Akihiro Miyauchi[b]

[a]*Hitachi Ltd., Research & Developing Group,*
832-2 Horiguchi, Hitachinaka, Ibaraki, Japan
[b]*Tokyo Medical and Dental University,*
Institute of Biomaterials and Bioengineering,
2-3-10 Kanda-Surugadai, Chiyodaku, Tokyo, Japan

mariko.miyazaki.jm@hitachi.com

14.1 Introduction

As pointed out by Vincent et al., the ways of building functional structures are different between biology and technology [1]. The surfaces of living matter have evolved into various functional 3D structures that are beyond human approach [2]. Biomimetics, that seeks sustainable solutions for practical problems by emulating nature's time-tested patterns, functions and strategies, has developed remarkably in recent years [3]. For example, sharkskin, as illustrated in Fig. 14.1, is covered with numerous small tooth-like elements, termed dermal denticles ("denticles" hereafter) [4, 5]. The hydrodynamic function of sharkskin has

---

Biomimetics: Connecting Ecology and Engineering by Informatics
Edited by Akihiro Miyauchi and Masatsugu Shimomura
Copyright © 2023 Jenny Stanford Publishing Pte. Ltd.
ISBN 978-981-4968-10-2 (Hardcover), 978-1-003-27717-0 (eBook)
www.jennystanford.com

been investigated for more than 30 years with the hypothesis that the microstructure of denticles, i.e., the minute projections, passively controls turbulent flow and reduces drag [6–13].

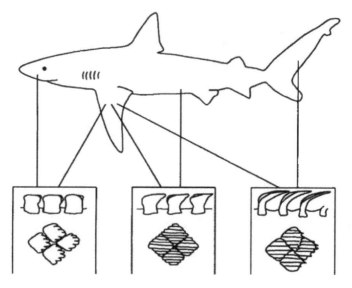

Figure 14.1 Examples of denticle structures at different position in sharkskin [4].

Sharkskin has been observed in two dimensions by using a scanning electron microscope (SEM), as shown in Fig. 14.2. However, a three-dimensional (3D) detailed view of the sharkskin structure has yet to be confirmed. Therefore, the "riblets," namely, the regular grooves with triangular or rectangular sections, have been studied both experimentally and computationally. Studies have confirmed that riblets are capable of reducing drag [14–21]. Actual denticles, however, in general demonstrate not simple riblet, but complicated 3D microstructures with a scale of less than 1 mm. Along with the recent rapid development in high-precision, high-performance 3D structural observation and analysis techniques for material surfaces, it has become possible to measure the 3D micro-surface structures of living matter such as sharks. Figure 14.3 shows the 3D structures of single denticles of a Blacktip reef shark observed by using a microfocus X-ray CT (Computed Tomography) measuring system.

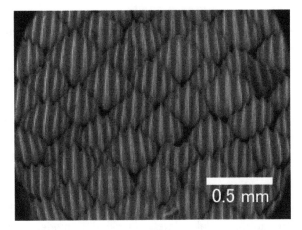

Figure 14.2 Sharkskin denticles of Blacktip reef shark observed by SEM.

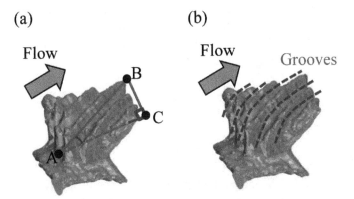

Figure 14.3 3D structures of single denticles of Blacktip reef shark. Structures of the denticles have two unique characteristics. (a) Sloping structure with large AOI (α). (b) Non-uniform grooves (with distinguished heights or spacing) in water flow direction.

From the 3D observation results, we proposed that denticle structures have two unique characteristics: a sloping structure with large angles of inclination (AOI) and grooves with distinguished heights or spacing in the water flow direction, namely non-uniform grooves [22, 23]. We clarified that the unique structures of the denticle (sloping structure and non-uniform grooves) generate complex, 3D local turbulent flows near the denticles, for example, a rising flow and multiple longitudinal vortices aligned with the water flow direction. We also proposed a prototype biomimetic riblet design inspired by sharkskin denticles and generated a similar flow to sharkskin from a 3D digitized structure of the denticles. We named a surface design method (namely observing living matters, understanding the mechanism of their functionality, and designing as structure that can reproduce the same function) "biomimetic design (BMD)." We applied the BMD to the diffuser vanes of a centrifugal compressor that reduced its efficiency, and confirmed the effect of the BMD on fluid performance [23, 24].

In recent years, denticles have been found to not only improve fluid properties but also provide an antibacterial effect. An antibacterial plate (Sharklet™) made of silicone elastomer imitating the structure of denticle was developed, and it was reported that this plate provided an antibacterial effect in various pathogenic microorganisms (*Staphylococcus aureus*, Methicillin-resistant *Staphylococcus aureus*, Pseudomonas aeruginosa, *Escherichia coli*, and vancomycin-resistant enterococci) [25, 26]. We considered that characteristic flow fields occurring on the sharkskin, i.e., rising flow and longitudinal vortices, suppress biofilm growth as well as improve fluid properties.

As the antibacterial effect in the surface of living matters, it was reported that the nanostructural surface of the wings of cicadas and dragonflies had an antibacterial property [27–29]. It was reported that a surface with nanostrucures which is significantly smaller than a bacterium had an effect of physically breaking the cell membranes of the bacteria [27]. However, it is considered that a nanostructural surface has only the initial antibacterial effect, as it does not suppress the growth of bacteria and the formation of a biofilm. We hypothesize that microstructural surface like denticles has a sustainable antibacterial effect achieved by suppressing the growth of the biofilm.

In this chapter, we introduce a biomimetic riblets design inspired by the antibacterial property of sharkskin denticles with microstructual surface with the biomimetic riblets inspired by sharkskin denticles [30].

14.2 Concept of Biofilm Growth Suppression

Biofilms clog the water intake of a power plant and filters of a seawater desalination plant, and it causes infections via a catheter in the medical field. In addition, metal corrosion due to sulfate-reducing bacteria in biofilms also causes many problems in areas of welding at plants.

Figure 14.4 shows the growth process of a biofilm. When a clean base material comes into contact with water, organic matter adheres immediately to the interface between water and the base material. It is interpreted as a conditioning layer for neutralizing the excess charge of the substrate and lowering the surface free energy [31, 32]. Even if a flow field is present, the water has viscosity, so the flow velocity on the surface of the substrate is zero and a so-called retention layer is formed, which makes it easy for bacteria to adhere. The bacteria that first adhere to the organic matter layer are called pioneer bacteria, and the first adhesion mechanism is electrostatic attraction or physical adhesion. In the attached bacteria, extracellular polysaccharide (EPS) adheres to the substrate, and the adhesion is stabilized. After that, the pioneer bacteria begin to grow and colonies coated with polysaccharides (glycocalyx) are formed [33]. Glycocalyx takes up other types of microbial cells and secondary colonies that metabolize the excretion of primary colonies consisting of pioneer bacteria are formed in the upper layer of primary colonies (pioneer colonies). This secondary colony adheres several days after primary colony formation [34]. Afterwards, microorganisms that metabolize the excretion of the secondary colonies adhere, and a multilayered colony structure is sequentially formed into a biofilm. The completed biofilm accumulates biochemical resources inside and completes a closed space in which water, excrement, nutrients, enzymes, oxygen, and so forth, traverse inside the film. As oxygen is unlikely to enter the biofilm, anaerobic bacteria can inhabit. Antibiotics used for biofilm removal, such as antiseptic solutions, only kill colonies of the outermost layer; the internal colony group does not die because it is self-sufficient in the closed space [35]. The once-formed biofilms are difficult to remove even by using a disinfectant solution, causing problems on all substrates that come into contact with water, such as in-hospital infections and filter clogging. As such, fundamental countermeasures do not exist. To suppress the growth of biofilms in water, suppressing the formation of an organic layer on the substrate is considered to be difficult because the surface energy of the substrate in water must be lowered. In subsequent colonization of pioneer bacteria, adhesion strength is considered to be weak, especially in the initial process. The basic concept is that the formation of primary colonies is inhibited by the self-breaking of pioneer bacteria colonies on the surface of the substrate, and the growth after secondary colonies does not occur.

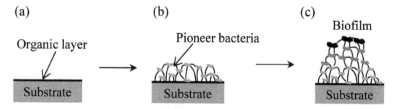

Figure 14.4 Growth mechanism of biofilm in water. (a) Organic layer coating on substrate. (b) Colony formation of pioneer-bacteria. (c) Additional colony formation on pioneer-bacteria colony.

Figure 14.5 shows a model of the substrate structure breaking the primary colony. This model applies a phenomenon in which microorganisms do not adhere to a sharkskin surface and breaks the primary colony by reproducing the 3D turbulent flow field near the denticles (the rising flow and multiple longitudinal vortices aligned with the water flow direction). This model exerts its effect in the presence of flow in the water.

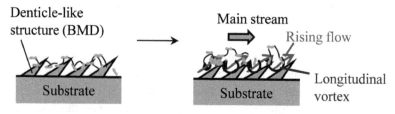

Figure 14.5 Schematic diagram of disrupting biofilm growth by breaking pioneer colony.

14.3 Preparation for the Culture Test of Bacteria

14.3.1 Fabrication of Test Sample

Samples used for the culture test of bacteria were prepared using nanoimprinting [36]. Figure 14.6 shows the fabrication process using nanoimprinting. A mold with a microstructure is attached to a resin film (Fig. 14.6a), and heat and pressure are applied to transfer the microstructure of the mold to the resin film (Fig. 14.6b). The mold is released from the resin film, and finally the resin film with the microstructure is fabricated (Fig. 14.6c).

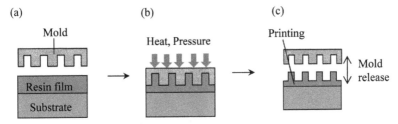

Figure 14.6 Method for fabricating resin sheet by nanoimprinting.

Figure 14.7 shows an overview of a mold in which a biomimetic-designed microstructure has been fabricated. A precision cutting method was used to fabricate the mold. Figure 14.7a shows a perspective view of the mold. The material of the mold is STAVAX, and its size is 20 × 20 × 10 mm. Figure 14.7b shows a top view of the mold. Seven types of biological deformed structure are fabricated in the mold. These structures were designed to reproduce the characteristic flow field (rising flow and longitudinal vortex) of the sharkskin as revealed in the previous study [22, 23]. Figure 14.7c shows a side view of the designed structure. An inclination of 27° is provided. Figure 14.7d shows a front view of the designed structure. Grooves are formed in which two triangles with different heights and widths are alternately arranged. The height h_1 and width w_1 of one triangle were fixed to 0.1 and 0.2 mm, respectively. The height h_2 and width w_2 of the other triangle were set to one of seven types shown in Table 14.1. The ratio of the heights (h_1/h_2) or widths (w_1/w_2) of the two triangles represents the magnitude of the non-uniformity of the groove.

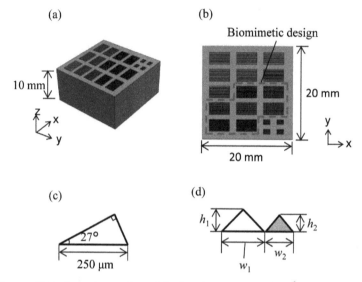

Figure 14.7 Overview of mold for biomimetic design fabrication. (a) Perspective view. (b) Top view. (c) Side view. (d) Front view.

Table 14.1 Triangle height and weight values of biomimetic design

No.	1	2	3	4	5	6	7
h_2 (mm)	0.01	0.02	0.033	0.05	0.1	0.2	0.2
w_2 (mm)	0.2	0.2	0.2	0.2	0.2	0.066	0.1

Procedures for fabricating a resin sheet from the mold are shown below. When transferring the structure from a metal mold directly to a resin sheet by nanoimprinting, incorrectly releasing the mold may result in the resin remaining in the mold, rendering the mold useless. Therefore, microstructures were processed on nickel by electroforming and microstructures were transferred to resin sheets by using this nickel plating foil for nanoimprint molds. As a result of examining the stability of the microstructure in advance, the ideal material of the resin was determined as cycloolefin polymer (COP). Figure 14.8 shows pictures of fabricated goods in processing nanoimprint.

Figure 14.8a shows the picture of the metal mold in which biomimetic-designed microstructure has been fabricated. Figure 14.8b shows the nickel-plating foil for nanoimprint molds. Figure 14.8c shows the COP sheet in which biomimetic-designed microstructure has been fabricated.

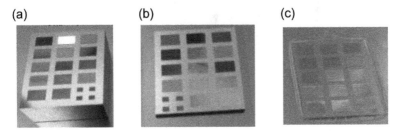

Figure 14.8 Pictures of fabricated goods in processing nanoimprint. (a) Metal mold. (b) Ni plated foil. (c) COP sheet fabricated biomimetic designs.

14.3.2 Method of Bacterial Culture

For the experiments in this chapter, a magnetic stirrer was used as a method to generate a flow in the culture solution in order to culture a bacterium in the presence of a flow. The flow state when the liquid was stirred with a stirrer was analyzed by computational fluid dynamics (CFD), and the design of the culture device and the test conditions were determined from the result of a CFD result.

Figure 14.9 shows the analysis model for designing the culture device. A stirrer bar with a diameter of 8 mm and a length of 40 mm was placed in the center of the bottom of a cylindrical area with a diameter of 85 mm and a height of 45 mm. The origin is at the center of the bottom, the x-axis is the direction in which the stirrer bar is placed, and the z-axis is the height direction of the cylindrical area. The bottom, side, and top of the culture device can be considered as locations for placing the test sample of bacterial culture. Therefore, we verified the flow state at each location when the stirrer bar was rotated at 1200 rpm to decide which location was appropriate for bacterial culture test.

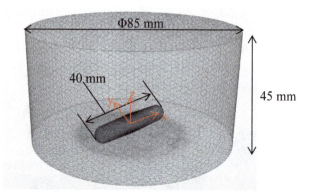

Figure 14.9 Analysis model for designing the culture device.

Figure 14.10 shows the flow state of the bottom surface of analysis area. Figures 14.10a,b show the velocity vector and velocity contour of x-y cross section (z = 0.3 mm). The candidate location for placing the test sample was indicated by black frames. As shown in Fig. 14.10, we found that a maximum flow velocity of about 0.5 m/s was generated near the center of the black frame, but a flow velocity near the wall surface was 0.1 m/s. The average swimming speed of a shark is 0.5 m/s and it is difficult to generate the same flow at the bottom.

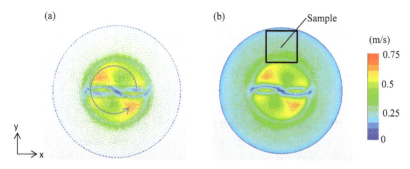

Figure 14.10 Flow state of the bottom surface. (a) Velocity vector of x-y cross section (z = 0.3 mm). (b) Velocity contour of x-y cross section (z = 0.3 mm).

Figure 14.11 shows the flow state of the top surface of analysis area. Figures 14.11a,b show the velocity vector and velocity contour of x-y cross section (z = 44 mm). The candidate location for placing the test sample was indicated by black frames. As shown in Fig. 14.11, we found that a large flow whose velocity was from 0.3 to 0.5 m/s was generated in the black frame area. However, a variation of velocity speed in the black frame area was large, that is, the velocity greatly varies depending on the location of the test sample.

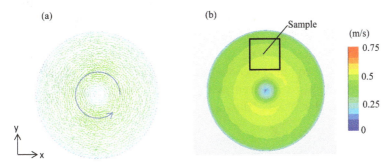

Figure 14.11 Flow state of the top surface. (a) Velocity vector of x-y cross section. (b) Velocity contour of x-y cross section.

Figure 14.12 shows the flow state of the side surface of analysis area. Figures 14.12a,b show the velocity vector and velocity contour of x-z cross section (y = 0 mm). The candidate location for placing the test sample was indicated by black line. As shown in Fig. 14.12, we found that a large flow whose velocity was about 0.5 m/s was generated in the black line area. Moreover, a variation of velocity speed in the black line area was small, that is, the velocity was almost same everywhere on the location of the test sample.

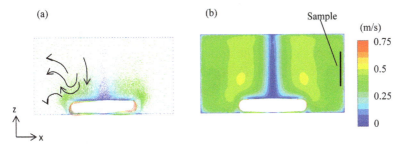

Figure 14.12 Flow state of the side surface. (a) Velocity vector of x-z cross section (y = 0 mm). (b) Velocity contour of x-z cross section (y = 0 mm).

From these results, we decided to place the test samples on the side surface of the container and set the rotation speed of the stirrer to 1200 rpm as the condition of the bacterial culture test.

Figure 14.13 shows the overview of the culture device. Figures 14.13a,b show the 3D design and the picture of culture device. A resin container for the test samples was placed in a glass Petri dish with an outer diameter of 90 mm, inner diameter of 85 mm and a height of 45 mm. In the container, grooves were fabricated at four places, and test samples were placed therein. The top of the container was covered with a glass round plate and were secured with screws. The culture test was conducted by placing the test bacterial solution in the culture device.

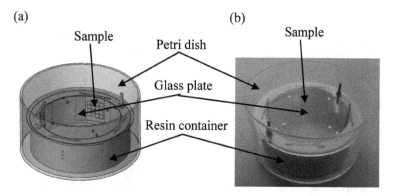

Figure 14.13 Overview of culture device. (a) 3D design. (b) Photograph.

14.3.3 Bacterial Culture Conditions

The bacterial culture conditions are shown in Table 14.2. *Staphylococcus aureus* subsp. aureus NBRC 15035 was used as the test bacteria. *Staphylococcus aureus* is a spherical bacterium having a diameter of about 0.9 μm. The suspension was cultured in a trypticase soy (SCD) broth medium to obtain a bacterial culture solution in which the number of test bacteria was 10^7–10^8/mL. As shown in Table 14.2, the medium was exchanged once a day. The bacteria were cultured in a state where a circulation was added using a stirrer, and samples were taken out on the fifth day from the start of the culture. The rotation speed of the stirrer was 1200 rpm. Figure 14.14 shows a photograph while the bacterial culture using the stirrer.

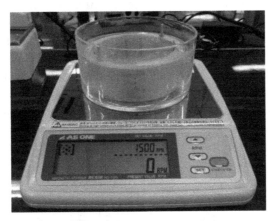

Figure 14.14 Photograph of bacterial culture using stirrer.

Table 14.2 Bacterial culture condition

Bacteria type	*Staphylococcus aureus* subsp. aureus NBRC 15035
Preparation of bacteria solution	The test bacteria are cultured in SCD broth medium at 37±1 °C for 18 to 24 h, and then suspended in SCD broth medium to prepare test bacteria in which the number of bacteria is 10^7 to 10^8 /mL.
Preparation of test samples	Sterilize test samples culturing equipment under high pressure steam sterilization (121 °C, 15 min), and place the test samples in a culture device. Add 300–350 mL of the bacterial solution, and incubate at 37±1 °C by stirring at 1200 rpm.
Test operation	Remove the test bacteria solution in the sample with a pipette once a day. Next, 300–350 mL of purified water is added, and the mixture is stirred for 1 minute at 1200 rpm, and the purified water is removed. After repeating this operation three times, add 300–350 mL of fresh SCD broth medium and recultivate at 37±1 °C.

14.3.4 Method of Coverage of Bacteria Quantification

To quantify the bacteria covering rate of the test samples, the samples taken out after culturing for five days were gram stained and observed with an optical microscope. Gram staining is a method for dyeing bacteria with pigments [37]. In this study, crystal violet was used as a staining solution. The test samples were immersed in a crystal violet solution for one minute and then stained by rinsing them with purified water. The covering rate of the bacteria was quantified by processing the optical microscope images obtained after dyeing. If more bacteria are attached to the test samples, more stains are observed, and the image appears darker. To quantify the covering ratio of bacteria, each pixel of the image was binarized in which black and white pixels represent areas where bacteria is and is not adhered, respectively and the covering of the bacteria is defined the following formula.

$$\text{Covering ratio of bacteria} = \frac{\text{Area of black area}}{\text{Total area of image}} \times 100(\%) \quad (14.1)$$

The density was quantified for each pixel of the image, and each pixel was set to black or white with the average value as a threshold value.

14.4 Evaluation of Antibacterial Effect by Biomimetics

Figure 14.15 shows an optical microscopic image (200 times) of the test samples stained with crystal violet. To determine the relationship between the height non-uniformity of the groove and the adhesion state of the bacteria, we reviewed the results of $h_1/h_2 = 1$ (No. 5 in Table 14.1), $h_1/h_2 = 5$ (No. 2 in Table 14.1) and $h_1/h_2 = 10$ (No. 1 in Table 14.1) among the seven grooved structures fabricated into the test samples.

Areas dyed purple in the image are where the bacteria adhered in the test sample. When $h_1/h_2 = 1$ where the grooves are uniform, the amount of adhered bacteria was high, and as the value of h_1/h_2 increased where the non-uniformity of the groove increases, the amount of bacteria adhered decreases.

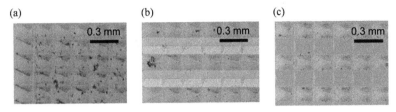

Figure 14.15 Microscope image of samples stained by crystal violet (200 times). (a) $h_1/h_2 = 1$. (b) $h_1/h_2 = 5$. (c) $h_1/h_2 = 10$.

Figure 14.16 shows the processed binarized image result of the optical microscope images shown in Fig. 14.15. Areas in which bacteria adhered are shown in black. Figure 14.17 shows a graph plotting the relationship between the groove height non-uniformity (h_1/h_2) and the coverage of the bacteria. When $h_1/h_2 = 1$ where grooves are uniform, the coverage is at the highest, and when h_1/h_2 increases, the coverage decreases as the groove non-uniformity increases. When $h_1/h_2 = 10$, the covering ratio decreased to 5%; a reduction of 10% compared with that when $h_1/h_2 = 1$. From the images shown in Fig. 14.16, the bacteria adhere to most of the area in the case of $h_1/h_2 = 1$. On the other hand, in the case of $h_1/h_2 = 5$ and $h_1/h_2 = 10$, the bacteria adhere in a band shape. The area with much bacteria adhered has a height h_2 and is the shallow groove, and the area with few bacteria adhered has a height h_1 and is the deep groove. If the non-uniformity of the groove is large, the flow speed increases at the shallow groove due to the occurrence of the longitudinal vortex and the bacteria attached to the surface are removed by the flow. As a result, formation of the biofilm was suppressed and the coverage of the bacteria was considered to be reduced.

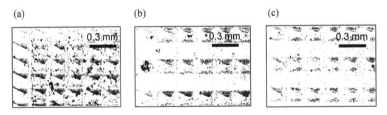

Figure 14.16 Image processing by binarization. (a) $h_1/h_2 = 1$. (b) $h_1/h_2 = 5$. (c) $h_1/h_2 = 10$.

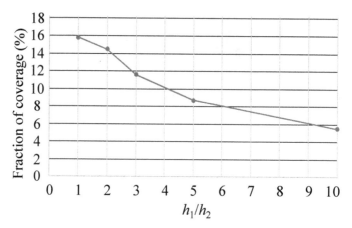

Figure 14.17 Relationship between non-uniformity and fraction of coverage.

14.5 Summary

In this chapter, we focused on the antibacterial effect of sharkskin, and evaluated the effect of suppressing biofilm growth with test samples of a fabricated biomimetic riblets design inspired by sharkskin denticles. Biomimetic designed structures to generate a similar flow to sharkskin were fabricated on COP sheets by nanoimprinting, and *Staphylococcus aureus* was cultured on these test samples in a state where circulation was added using a stirrer. Our results indicate that as the non-uniformity of the grooves increases, the bacteria adhering to the surface is removed due to the effect of the longitudinal vortex generated on the sharkskin, and the coverage ratio of bacteria is reduced.

The nanostructural surface of the wings of cicadas and dragonflies has the effect of antibacterial property by physically breaking the cell membranes of the bacteria. On the other hand, the microstructual surface inspired by sharkskin denticles has the effect of antibacterial property by suppressing the growth of bacteria and the formation of biofilm. Therefore, the microstructual surface is considered to have sustainable antibacterial effect compared to the nanostructural surface.

The surfaces of living matter have evolved into various functional 3D structures that are beyond human approach. If we design an artificial surface structure while understanding functions and strategies of living matters, we can design to specifically improve only functions required for engineering products. Therefore, it is possible to exert the performance superior to the functions that living matters originally have. This is the excellent advantage of about the surface design using BMD.

Acknowledgments

The authors thank Mr. Tokui of Tempstaff for experiments and discussion; Prof. Shimomura and Dr. Hirai of Chitose Institute of Science and Technology for fruitful discussion; and Drs. Tomita and Sato of Churaumi Aquarium for supplying shark skin specimens. A part of this chapter was supported by the New Energy Development Organization (NEDO) of Japan.

References

1. Vincent, J. F. V., Bogatyreva, O. A., Bogatyrev, N. R., Bowyer, A., and Pahl, A. K. (2006). Biomimetics: its practice and theory. *J. R. Soc. Interface*, **3**, 471–482.

2. Bhushan, B. (2012). Bioinspired structured surfaces. *Lamgmuir*, **28**, 1698–1714.

3. Liu, H., Nakata, T., Li, G., and Kolomenskiy, D. (2017). Unsteady bio-fluid dynamics in flying and swimming. *Acta Mechanica Sinica*, **33**, 663–684.

4. Wen, L., Weaver, J. C., and Lauder, G. V. (2014). Biomimetic shark skin: design, fabrication and hydrodynamic function. *J. Exp. Biol.*, **217**, 1656–1666.

5. Kemp, N. E. (1999). *Integumentary System and Teeth in Sharks, Skates, and Rays: The Biology of Elasmobranch Fishes* (Hamlet W. C., ed), Johns Hopkins University Press, Baltimore.

6. Meyer, W., and Seegers, U. (2012). Basics of skin structure and function in elasmobranchs: a review. *J. Fish Biol.*, **80**, 1940–1967.

7. Castro, J. I. (2011). *The Sharks of North America*, Oxford University Press.

8. Reif, W. E., and Dinkelacker, A. (1982). Hydrodynamics of the squamation in fast swimming sharks. *Neues Jahrb. Geol. Palaontol. Abh.*, **164**, 184–187.

9. Reif, W. E. (1985). Squamation and Ecology of Sharks, Frankfurt am Main: Senckenbergische Naturforschende Gesellschaft.

10. Bechert, D. W., Bruse, M., Hage, W., van der Hoeven J., and Hoppe, G. (1997). Experiments on drag-reducing surfaces and their optimization with an adjustable geometry. *J. Fluid Mech.*, **338**, 59–87.

11. Bechert, D. W., Bruse, M., and Hage, W. (2000). Experiments with three-dimensional riblets as an idealized model of sharkskin. *Exp. Fluids*, **28**, 403–412.

12. Lang, A. W., Motta, P., Hueter, R., Habegger, M., and Farhana, A. (2011). Shark skin separation control mechanisms. *J. Mar. Technol. Soc.*, **45**, 208–215.

13. Walsh, M. J. (1980). Drag characteristics of V-Groove and transverse curvature riblets. *AIAA J.*, **72**, 168–184.

14. Walsh, M. J. (1983). Riblets as a viscous drag reduction technique. *AIAA J.*, **21**, 485–486.

15. Vukoslavcevic, P., Wallace, J. M., and Balint, J. I. (1992). Viscous drag reduction using streamwise-aligned riblets. *AIAA J.*, **30**, 1119–1122.

16. Choi, H., Moin, P., and Kim, J. (1993). Direct numerical simulation of turbulent flow over riblets. *J. Fluid Mech.*, **255**, 503–539.

17. Park, S. R. (1994). Flow alteration and drag reduction by riblets in a turbulent boundary layer. *AIAA J.*, **32**, 31–38.

18. Lee, S. J., and Lee, S. H. (2001). Flow field analysis of a turbulent boundary layer over a riblet surface. *Exp. Fluids*, **30**, 153–166.

19. Dean, B., and Bhushan, B. (2010). Shark skin surfaces for fluid-drag reduction in turbulent flow: a review. *Phil. Trans. R. Soc.*, **A368**, 4775–4806.

20. Buttner, C. C., and Shulz, U. (2011). Shark skin inspired riblet structures as aerodynamically optimized high temperature coatings for blades of aeroengines. *Smart Materials and Structures*, **20**, 094016 (9pp).

21. Luo, Y., Liu, Y., Zhang, D., and Ng, E. Y. K. (2014). Influence of morphology for drag reduction effect of sharkskin surface. *J. Mech. Med. Biol.*, **14**, 1450029 (16pp).

22. Miyazaki, M., Hirai, Y., Moriya, H., Shimomura, M., Miyauchi, A., and Liu, H. (2018). Biomimetic riblets inspired by sharkskin denticles: digitizing, modeling and flow simulation. *Bionic Engineering*, **15**, 999–1011.

23. Miyauchi, A. (2018). 3D Modeling of shark skin and prototype diffuser for fluid control, in *Indusrial Biomimetics* (Miyauchi, A. and Shimomura, M., ed), Chapter 1, Jenny Stanford Publishing.

24. Miyazaki, M., Hirai, Y., Moriya, H., Shimomura, M., Miyauchi, A., and Liu, H. (2018). Biomimetic design inspired sharkskin denticles and modeling of diffuser for fluid control. *J. Photopolym. Sci. Technol.*, **31**, 133–138.

25. Chung, K. K., Schumacher, J. F., Sampson, E. M., Burne, R. A., Antonelli, P. J., and Brennan, A. B. (2007). Impact of engineered surface microtopography on biofilm formation of *Staphylococcus aureus*. *Biointerphases*, **2**, 89–94.

26. Reddy, S. T., Chung, K. K, McDaniel, C. J., Darouiche, R. O., Landman, J., and Brennan, A. B. (2011). Micropatterned surfaces for reducing the risk of catheter-associated urinary tract infection: an in vitro study on the effect of sharklet micropatterned surfaces to inhibit bacterial colonization and migration of uropathogenic *Escherichia coli. J. Endourol.*, **25**, 1547–1552.

27. Ivanova, E. P., Hasen, J., Webb, H. K., Gervinskas, G., Juodkazis, S., Truong, V. K., Wu, A. H. F., Lamb, R. N., Baulin, V. A., Watson, G. S., Watson, J. A., Mainwaring, D. E., and Crawford, R. J. (2013). Bactericidal activity of black silicon. *Nat. Commun.*, **4**, 2838–2845.

28. Hasan, J., Webb, H. K., Truong, V. K., Pogodin, S., Baulin, V. A., Watson, G. S., Watson, J. A., Crawford, R. J., and Ivanova, E. P. (2013). Selective bactericidal activity of nanopatterned superhydrophobic cicada *Psaltoda claripennis* wing surfaces. *Appl. Microbiol. Biotechnol.*, **97**, 9257–9262.

29. Nakade, K., Sagawa, T., Kojima, H., Shimizu, T., Shingubara, S., and Ito, T. (2019). Single cell/real-time imaging of bactericidal effect on the nano-structural surface. *Material Today: Proceedings*, **7**, 497–500.

30. Miyazaki, M., Moriya, H., M., and Miyauchi, A. (2019). Biomimetic design inspired sharkskin denticles for growth suppression of biofilm. *J. Photopolym. Sci. Technol.*, **32**, 295–301.

31. Mittelman, M. W. (1985). Biological fouling of purified-water systems: part 1, bacterial growth and replication. *Microcontamination*, **3**, 51–55.

32. Mittelman, M. W. (1985). Biological fouling of purified-water systems: part 2, detection and enumeration. *Microcontamination*, **3**, 42–58.

33. Mayette, D. C. (1992). The existence and significance of biofilms in water, *Water Rev.*, Water Quality Research Council, Lisle Il, pp. 1–3.

34. Borenstein, S. B. (1994). *Microbiologically Influenced Corrosion Handbook*, Industrial Press Inc., New York.

35. Coghlan, A. (1996). Slime city. *New Scientist*, **15**, 32–36.

36. Miyauchi, A. (2019). *Nanoimprinting and Its Applications*, Jenny Stanford Publishing.

37. Wilhelm, M. J., Sheffield, J. B., Sharifian, Gh. M., Wu, Y., Spahr, C., Gonella, G., Xu, B., and Dai, H. L. (2015). Gram's stain does not cross the bacterial cytoplasmic membrane. *ACS Chem. Biol.*, **10**, 1711–1717.

Index

absorption 188–189, 203, 275, 285

acetabulum 150, 163–164, 177

actuators 4, 76–77, 179–180

adhesion 47, 244, 251–252, 280, 291, 301

adsorption 174, 176–177, 244

adsorption strength 175–177

agricultural ecosystems 105–106, 108, 110, 112, 114, 116, 118, 120

agriculture 5, 13–14, 16–17, 243

air-liquid interfacial areas 211, 214

air–water interface 220, 222, 229

algorithms 59–60

amino acids 245–246, 263

antennae (insects) 119, 121

anti-barnacle settlement activity 140–141, 219

anti-biofouling effects 129–130, 132–136, 138, 140, 142, 144

antibacterial characteristics 172–173

antibacterial effect 300, 310–312
  evaluation of 310–311

antifouling 33–36, 46, 129, 132–133, 135–136, 140–142, 284–285, 288–289, 292, 294

Aphididae 107–108

aphids 244–248, 250, 254
  gall-inducing 246–247
  liquid marbles fabricated by 245, 247, 249–250, 254

apoptosis 98–99, 101

aqueous dispersion 250–251, 267, 273

artificial melanin-based structural color materials 261–262, 264, 266, 268, 270, 272, 274

asymmetry 74, 85–87

bacteria 171–172, 300–301, 308–312
  culture test of 303, 305, 307, 309
  pioneer 301–302

bacterial culture 305, 308–309

barnacle cypris larvae 132, 134–135, 143

barnacle growth 138, 140

barnacle growth inhibition 138–139, 217

barnacle larval settlements 130, 133–135, 142–143

barnacle settlements 136, 138, 141

barnacles 130–133, 136, 138–141, 144
  settled 136–138, 143

basal adhesive plaque
  bio-interfaces 138–139

basal plates 138–140

beetles 106–107, 109–111, 191
  group-living 107
  jewel 192, 194, 196, 262
  scarab 192–193

BID, *see* biology-inspired design

bile 280, 285, 290

Index

bile duct stent having antifouling properties 279–280, 282, 284, 286, 288, 290, 292, 294
bile ducts 292–294
biliary stents 279–280, 284–285, 288–289, 292–294
bio-organisms 54, 57, 61, 64–65
bio-TRIZ 75–76, 83
biocompatible material 4, 9–10, 12–13, 20, 71, 275
biodiversity 2
biofilm 300–302, 311–312
biofilm-inspired sharkskin denticles 297–298, 300, 302, 304, 306, 308, 310, 312
biofunctions 70–71, 75, 80–81, 88
biological organisms 30, 35, 54–55
biology-inspired design (BID) 29–31, 47–48
biomimetic design 261, 304
biomimetic devices 149–150, 152, 154, 156, 158, 160, 162, 164, 166, 168, 170, 172, 174, 176, 178, 180, 182
biomimetic information 83
biomimetic methodology 30
biomimetic perspective 92
biomimetic products 70, 80–81, 84–85, 87
biomimetic riblets 300
biomimetic structure 289–294
biomimetic technology 1, 6–8, 17–18, 20–21
biomimetics
  applications of 19, 70, 72, 105
  knowledge infrastructure for 28–29, 31–33, 35
  new developments in 56
  ontology 25, 27–28, 37, 39, 42–43, 45
  research 25, 149–150

social implementation of 3, 21, 24
technologies 21, 282–283
thesauri 35, 38, 41
biomimetics databases 35–37, 39–40, 42
biotechnology 3
BioTRIZ 29–30
blacktip reef shark 298–299
bouncing 207–208, 220, 226–238
bouncing raindrops on lotus leaf 220–221, 223, 225, 227, 229
bugs 106–107, 109, 111
butterflies 192, 194, 197, 262

$CaCO_3$ particles 250–252
cancerous growth 96, 99–100
Cassie–Baxter state 210, 219–220, 222, 235
cell death 97–98
Cerambycidae 107–108, 110
chordotonal organs, femoral 108–109
cicadas 65, 149–150, 170–171, 300, 312
Coleoptera 106–107
coleopteran families 107, 110
colloidal crystal structure 264, 269
colloidal crystals 195–196, 262, 264, 267
colloidal particles 195, 199, 264, 271
colonies, primary 301–302
color 44, 74, 188–189, 191–201, 248, 261–262, 265, 268–269, 273
  pigment 261
color materials
  artificial structural 264
  fibrous structural 273–274

coloration 189, 264, 269–271
communication 5, 29, 32, 106, 110, 119
  sexual 106–107, 110
  social 106–107
  vibrational 110
consumer products 6, 14, 17
Cydnidae 107–108
cypris larvae 131–132, 143

DAE, *see* diarylethene
daidzein 114–115
deep learning technologies 57, 60
denticles 297–300, 302
diarylethene (DAE) 215, 220–221, 223–224, 226, 230–231, 236
diffraction 188, 190–191, 196, 198, 201, 262
diffraction grating 188, 190, 261, 264
disaster rescue robot 5, 13–15
diseases, lifestyle-related 92–93, 95, 97
dopamine 263–265, 270–271
double-roughness structure (DRS) 207–208, 215, 219–221, 225–228
dragonflies 71, 86–87, 170, 192, 194, 300, 312
droplets, macroscopic 208, 220, 229–230, 238
DRS, *see* double-roughness structure
duodenum 280, 285, 291
dynamic pressure 208, 220, 225–226, 229–230, 238

earthworms 33–34

EBSs, *see* endoscopic biliary stent
ecology 130, 243
ecosystems 2–3
elastic modulus 134–135
elasticity 133–135
electronics 85, 87, 250
endoscopic biliary stent (EBSs) 280–281
energy
  adhesion 208, 218, 230, 234–236, 238
  dissipation 208, 230, 234–236, 238
  pinning 210, 214, 217
  potential 217, 238
energy transfer 189, 193
engineering problems 26, 72, 80, 85
Eriosoma moriokense 246–249
ESR, *see* evolutionarily stable region
evolutionarily stable region (ESR) 102–103

feeding damage 112, 114
fine-processing technology 150
fisheries 5, 13–14, 16–17
formononetin 114–115
function-oriented approach 70, 83–88
functional agglomeration 103

geckos 149, 174–177
  feet 42, 174
  footpads of 149–150, 174–175
gravity 168, 170
gripping 166–170, 178

hawks 86–87, 102–103
Hemiptera 106–107
hemipteran families 106–107
Himeshirazu 113, 115–117
honeydew 245–247, 249
human eye 263, 267
hydrogels 129–130, 132–138, 143
  double-network 134, 136
  swelling degrees of 135
hydrophobic materials 4, 10,
  20–21, 71

IAC100 112–118
insect pest control 5, 13–14, 16–17
insects 7, 24, 66, 86, 106, 108,
  111–112, 118–119, 170, 207,
  230, 243, 262
interactions
  biological 105–106, 108, 110,
    112, 114, 116, 118, 120
  predator–prey 106–107
  vibrational 106–107, 109, 111
International Standard
    Organization (ISO) 2, 27,
    70, 80
inventive problem-solving 70, 72,
  74, 76, 78–84, 86, 88
ISO, *see* International Standard
    Organization
ISO specifications 70, 80, 85, 88

Japan Patent Office (JPO) 4–5, 71
Japanese elm 246–247
JPO, *see* Japan Patent Office

labrum 155–159, 162
Laplace pressure 208, 220, 222,
  224–226, 229, 238

larvae 107–108, 110, 112, 114,
  116, 130
light emission 188, 192
light scattering 263, 265, 267, 272
light wavelength 195, 197, 199,
  264
Linked Open Data (LOD) 37, 40
liquid crystal 191–192, 195–196
liquid marble 244, 250
liquid marbles 244–245, 247–250,
  254–255
LOD, *see* Linked Open Data
lotus 33, 36, 42, 70, 244, 279, 285
lotus effect 171, 208, 210, 213,
  215, 238
lotus leaf 33–34, 207–208, 213,
  215–221, 223, 225–227,
  229–230, 238
  bouncing behaviors of water
    droplets on 220–221
  structured surfaces mimicking
    229

macrotrichia 230–231, 234
melanin 196, 262–263, 270, 275
  artificial 262–263, 265–275
  natural 263–264, 274–275
membranes, porous 78–79
MEMS, *see* microelectromechanical
    systems
microelectromechanical systems
    (MEMS) 150–151, 153
microneedle 152–153, 158–162
  for drawing blood 154–155, 157,
    159, 161
  hollow 159–160, 162
  stainless 163
microstructures 70, 150, 262–263,
  270–271, 298, 303–304
  biomimetic-designed 303, 305

mimicking 150, 154, 157, 162,
172, 174, 177–178, 182, 244,
274, 283
mimicking mosquitoes 154–155,
157, 159, 161
Monochamus alternatus 108–111
morpho butterfly 196–197, 199
single colored structural color
197, 199
mosquito needle 155
mosquito proboscis 151, 155,
157, 163
mosquitoes 150–152, 154–160,
162, 230
moths 70, 118, 120–121, 203
multilayer film 191, 194–196,
199–200, 262
multipillar surface 222–223, 234

nanoimprinting 154, 291,
303–304, 312
natural principle 83, 87
nature 6, 18, 49, 66, 75, 80, 84–85,
196–197, 244, 246, 254–255,
262–263, 265, 275, 283
necrosis 98, 101
needle-shaped crystals 215, 224,
227, 232, 236
needle-shaped structures
207–208, 224
needles 151, 154–161, 227–229,
231
hollow 158, 162–163
painless 149–150, 154–155
Nitidulidae 107, 110
norepinephrine 270–271
nutrients 245–246, 301

octopus acetabulum 163–165,
167, 169, 171, 173

OET, *see* Ontology-Enhanced
Thesaurus
oil droplet 284
oil repellency 279, 283–284, 287
olfactory receptor neurons (ORNs)
119–120
olfactory receptors (insect)
119–120
ontologies 26–27, 29–31, 34, 38,
40–47, 49, 56
functional 43
upper 27, 44
Ontology-Enhanced Thesaurus
(OET) 25–29, 31–46, 48–49
ontology exploration tool 39–40
organisms
marine 129, 141
natural 54, 244
ORNs, *see* olfactory receptor
neurons
osteoporosis 95–96

PAAm, *see* poly(acrylamide)
PAMPS, *see* poly(2- acrylamide–2-
methyl-1-propanesulfonate)
PDMS, *see* poly(dimethylsiloxane)
peacock feathers 262, 269, 271
Pentatomidae 106–107
pest control 109–111
pheromone blend 118–121
phloem sap 245–246
pigeons 102–103, 192
pigs, bile ducts of 291, 293–294
pinning effect 208, 210, 213–214,
223, 238
plant protection 105–107, 109,
111
poly(2-acrylamide–2-methyl-1-
propanesulfonate) (PAMPS)
134, 136
poly(acrylamide) (PAAm) 134,
136–137, 140

poly(dimethylsiloxane) (PDMS)
138–139, 141–142, 160, 199
poly(vinyl alcohol) (PVA)
133–134, 136
polydopamine 262–267, 274–275
polystyrene 133–134, 138,
267–268
predators 106–108, 208, 249
pressure-sensitive adhesives
(PSAs) 243–244, 246, 248,
250–254
problem-oriented approach
82–83, 85, 88
problem-solving principles 73,
75, 81
PSAs, see pressure-sensitive
adhesives
PVA, see poly(vinyl alcohol)
PVA hydrogel 136–138

raindrops 208, 220, 225, 230
randomness 199–200
refractive index 191, 193, 196,
201–202, 261, 264, 272
rolling behavior 208, 215, 218

SAMs, see self-assembled
monolayers
sandfish 35–36
SDGs, see Sustainable Development
Goals
self-assembled monolayers (SAMs)
132–133
self-repairing material 4, 9–10,
12, 20
sensors 4, 71, 201–203, 245
sensory neurons 108–109

sessile organisms 129–130,
132–134, 136–138, 140–144
sex pheromone receptors
119–121
sex pheromones 118–120
sharkskin 244, 297–298, 300, 303,
312
sharkskin denticles 300, 312
shear stress 249, 251–253
Si_3N_4 199
silicone elastomers 129–130,
132–133, 138, 141, 143, 300
microstructured 140–141, 143,
219
single-roughness structures (SRS)
215–216, 220, 226
SiO_2 172–173, 199–200
skin 151, 154, 156, 262, 275, 284
artificial 160
snail shells 279, 282–286
structure 283
snails 36, 282–284
soap bubbles 190–192, 197, 261
soft materials 129–130, 132–136,
138–140, 142–144, 217
antifouling properties of 130,
132
soybean 114, 117
soybean leaf trichomes 112–113,
115, 117
Spodoptera litura 112–118
SRS, see single-roughness
structures
stent 280, 286–287, 291–292, 294
metallic 280
plastic 134, 138–140, 280, 282
stent-occlusion 279–280
stinging motion 155–156, 160
structural color 61, 70, 187–198,
200, 202–204, 261–267,
269–275

angular dependence of 269
applications of 192–193
non-iridescent 269
visible 196, 271
structural color materials 4, 262, 264–267, 269, 271, 273–275
structural color pellets 268–269
structural color visibility 266, 273
structural coloration 262, 265, 271, 275
structural colors 197, 267, 274
structured surfaces 207–208, 210, 212, 214, 216, 218, 220, 222, 224, 226, 228–238
structures
amorphous 269
bellows 168–170
biological 150–151
denticle 298–299
double-roughness 207, 215, 219–221, 225–226, 228
flat 78–79
nanopillar 170–171, 173
nanoscale 283, 286
opal 191
porous 77, 79
sloping 299
super-hydrophilic 280, 282–283
two-layer 174, 177
suction 164–165, 170, 177–180
sugars 245–246
surface area 85, 88, 203, 209
surface microstructures 142
surface pits 142
surfaces
double-roughness 221, 223–225
hydrophilic 134, 212–213, 238
microstructual 300, 312
nanostructural 300, 312
stepped 168
Sustainable Development Goals (SDGs) 76, 80, 84–85

Tamahomare 112, 114–116
Tenebrionidae 106–108
termite wing 208, 220, 230–231, 238
dual surface structure mimicking 230
Terpnosia nigricosta 65–66
Theory of Inventive Problem Solving (TRIZ) 69–70, 72–76, 79, 83, 85
thermodynamics 208, 210, 238
thin film 74, 79, 85, 191, 195, 261, 265
three-dimensional laser lithographic system 152–153, 159–160
TiO_2 191, 200
tonic immobility 108, 110
trichomes 112–118
TRIZ, *see* Theory of Inventive Problem Solving

ultra-high-precision three-dimensional processing 150–151, 153
urban planning 91–92, 94, 96, 98–102
UV irradiation 215–216

vacuum suction gripper 150, 163, 165, 167, 169, 171, 173
vibration exciters 109, 111
vibrations
artificial 110–111
low-frequency 110
mechanical 74, 77

water 33–34, 78, 168, 170, 225, 229, 235, 238, 254, 265, 279, 283–285, 287, 289, 301–302
purified 309–310
water droplets 207–209, 211, 213–217, 220–223, 225–229, 231, 233, 236
water repellence 33
Wenzel state 209–210, 219, 229
wettability 143
wetting 207–214, 217–219, 222, 230, 235, 238, 245

on structured surfaces 207–208, 210, 212, 214, 216, 218, 220, 222, 224, 228, 230, 232, 234, 236, 238
windmills 85–87
wings 65, 86–87, 149, 171, 197, 230–231, 262

zoospores 132–133

Printed in the USA
CPSIA information can be obtained
at www.ICGtesting.com
LVHW010933190324
774517LV00003BA/241